Managing PTSD for Health and Social Care Professionals

Dr Jan Smith

T0271791

Overcoming Common Problems Series

Selected titles

A full list of titles is available from Sheldon Press on our website at
www.sheldonpress.co.uk

The A to Z of Eating Disorders
Emma Woolf

Autism and Asperger Syndrome in Adults
Dr Luke Beardon

Chronic Pain the Drug-free Way
Phil Sizer

Coping with Aggressive Behaviour
Dr Jane McGregor

Coping with Diverticulitis
Peter Cartwright

Coping with Headaches and Migraine
Alison Frith

**Coping with the Psychological Effects of
Illness**
Dr Fran Smith, Dr Carina Eriksen and Professor
Robert Bor

Dementia Care: A guide
Christina Macdonald

Depression and Anxiety the Drug-free Way
Mark Greener

Depressive Illness: The curse of the strong
Dr Tim Cantopher

Dr Dawn's Guide to Sexual Health
Dr Dawn Harper

Dr Dawn's Guide to Toddler Health
Dr Dawn Harper

Dr Dawn's Guide to Your Baby's First Year
Dr Dawn Harper

**Dying for a Drink: All you need to know to
beat the booze**
Dr Tim Cantopher

**The Empathy Trap: Understanding antisocial
personalities**
Dr Jane McGregor and Tim McGregor

**Everything Your GP Doesn't Have Time to Tell
You about Alzheimer's**
Dr Matt Piccaver

**Everything Your GP Doesn't Have Time to Tell
You about Arthritis**
Dr Matt Piccaver

**Gestational Diabetes: Your survival guide to
diabetes in pregnancy**
Dr Paul Grant

The Heart Attack Survival Guide
Mark Greener

The Holistic Guide for Cancer Survivors
Mark Greener

**Hope and Healing after Stillbirth and New
Baby Loss**
Professor Kevin Gournay and Dr Brenda Ashcroft

How to Stop Worrying
Dr Frank Tallis

IBS: Dietary advice to calm your gut
Alex Gazzola and Julie Thompson

Living with Angina
Dr Tom Smith

Living with Multiple Sclerosis
Mark Greener

Living with Tinnitus and Hyperacusis
Dr Laurence McKenna, Dr David Baguley and Dr
Don McFerran

**Mental Health in Children and Young People:
Spotting symptoms and seeking help early**
Dr Sarah Vohra

The Multiple Sclerosis Diet Book
Tessa Buckley

**Parenting Your Disabled Child: The first three
years**
Margaret Barrett

Sleep Better: The science and the myths
Professor Graham Law and Dr Shane Pascoe

Stress-related Illness
Dr Tim Cantopher

**Taming the Beast Within: Understanding
personality disorder**
Professor Peter Tyrer

Therapy Pets: A guide
Jill Eckersley

**Toxic People: Dealing with dysfunctional
relationships**
Dr Tim Cantopher

Treating Arthritis: The drug-free way
Margaret Hills and Christine Horner

Treating Arthritis Diet Book
Margaret Hills

Understanding Hoarding
Jo Cooke

Vertigo and Dizziness
Jaydip Ray

**Wellbeing: Body confidence, health and
happiness**
Emma Woolf

**Your Guide for the Cancer Journey: Cancer
and its treatment**
Mark Greener

Lists of titles in the Mindful Way and Sheldon Short Guides series are also available from Sheldon Press.

Overcoming Common Problems

Managing PTSD for Health and Social Care Professionals

Help for the Helpers

DR JAN SMITH

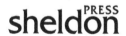

First published by Sheldon Press in 2022
An imprint of John Murray Press
A division of Hodder & Stoughton Ltd,
An Hachette UK company

This paperback edition published in 2022

1

This book is for information or educational purposes only and is not intended to act as a substitute for medical advice or treatment. Any person with a condition requiring medical attention should consult a qualified medical practitioner or suitable therapist.

A CIP catalogue record for this title is available from the British Library

Trade Paperback ISBN 978 1529 37105 5
eBook ISBN 978 1529 37106 2

Typeset by KnowledgeWorks Global Ltd.

Printed and bound in Great Britain by Clays Ltd, Elcograf S.p.A.

John Murray Press policy is to use papers that are natural, renewable and recyclable products and made from wood grown in sustainable forests. The logging and manufacturing processes are expected to conform to the environmental regulations of the country of origin.

John Murray Press
Carmelite House
50 Victoria Embankment
London EC4Y 0DZ

www.sheldonpress.co.uk

Author's note

You will have your own reasons why you've picked up this book to read. I urge you to read it with care and safety. Some of the contents of this book might feel difficult for you to read. There are a number of exercises you are invited to complete throughout the chapters. Please take care when you are engaging with these. Check in at regular times with yourself: how you're breathing, whether your heart's beating faster, or you're beginning to feel overwhelmed. You can switch off from it at any time by taking a break and putting this book down. Indeed, I would encourage you to do this.

Throughout the book, I've tried to use the terminology 'helping professions' to acknowledge the range of health and social care staff who work in challenging environments and are vulnerable to being emotionally impacted by their work. This book is also for anyone in management or leadership positions working in or alongside staff from these sectors.

The book is divided into two parts. The first part focuses on developing your emotional language through learning how to create healthy habits and maintaining them and a range of evidence-based practices to prevent the impact of trauma, compassion fatigue, burnout and moral injury. The second part explores the barriers to reaching out for help and accessing routine and professional support.

Acknowledgements

No book exists solely because of the author, and this book is here because of many people. To the numerous staff over the years who have reached out to me, brought me into their world and allowed me to walk alongside them on their journey of healing. For those who trusted me when I reached in – thank you for taking a risk with me. I have learned so much from you all over the years. I have been inspired by many professionals who I've had the pleasure to work with and been supervised by. My leadership and coaching work has provided the opportunity for me to work with some truly exceptional leaders, who 'show up' in the service of those they lead.

To my friends, who never fail to bring humour and fun times when I need it the most – thank you. Two of my biggest champions: Mark and Mike. Your belief in what I can achieve and the support that you give me, in anything I ever set out to do, are bountiful. For my parents, who taught me from an early age what it means to see the 'human' in every interaction I have. This teaching has been invaluable for me, both personally and professionally. Last, but by no means least, my cherubs, who challenge my thinking and continue to teach me what it means to be mindful, forgiving and kind. I am truly grateful to you all.

Contents

Disclaimer

The pages in this book are filled with evidence-based practices that have been shown to be effective in supporting individuals in order to optimize their mental wellbeing or seek professional support. Research is just that; it is not facts. We are all different, and so what might work for one person will be less helpful for others. This book is not intended to replace any current support you are receiving. Instead, it is here to inspire you to begin thinking about how you can strengthen the relationship you have with yourself and implement ways to care for your mental wellbeing while working in a challenging role.

I hope you find it helpful and that you find something here that resonates with you.

About the author

Dr Jan Smith is a Chartered Psychologist, Executive Coach and Director of Healthy You Ltd. For over 15 years she has worked with individuals and organisations on creating ways to prevent and manage the impact of psychological trauma, moral injury or stress. Jan has particular expertise in creating psychologically safe and positive working cultures in organizations. In the UK, she is the Clinical Lead for the national birth trauma campaign Make Birth Better. In addition to being an expert advisor on how to create trauma-informed services and psychologically safe organizations, Jan provides consultancy services across a number of industries, including the aviation sector, and is Head of Wellbeing and Clinical Services at Kura Human Factors. She holds a research post at Sheffield Hallam University.

Introduction

If you've picked up this book, then it could be that you are seeking to understand better the role that psychological trauma can have on helping professionals, and to find ways to feel relief from your symptoms. Dealing with a traumatic event can feel incredibly isolating and frightening, and can negatively affect relationships and working life, as well as the sense of who you are. You are not alone: traumatic events happen to individuals worldwide, with global prevalence rates as high as 37 per cent. Many affected learn how to recover and carry on with their lives.

Human beings suffer. We can't get away from the fact that we will be impacted by physical and mental illness at some point in our lifetime. However, believing this can be difficult because it also means accepting that we are vulnerable, and are subject to experiencing conditions that afflict the general population, such as depression, anxiety and trauma. Having a strong sense of identity, holding on to work-related values, and contributing to a professional culture, are all factors which could make us excel in our careers. However, what if these factors stopped us from reaching out for support when we needed help the most? I often witness staff feeling ashamed for not being able to 'just get on with things' when they sit in the role of the patient or client.

Meeting others' needs, caring for them with compassion, and helping others to maintain boundaries is often at the core of what we do. Furthermore, we understand that there are often wide-ranging and complex factors that impact our patients' or clients' health and wellbeing. However, we can find it challenging to recognize these factors affecting our own wellbeing and tend not to show ourselves the same care and compassion we so readily show others.

1

The cost of caring for helpers

Everyone experiences stress, to varying degrees, and how someone responds to that stress is often individual. As a society, we expect that people feel stressed, so there's a level of adjustment, tolerance and acceptance of this. Stress reactions can be the first indication of emotional trauma. However, terms like 'stressful', 'traumatic', 'compassion fatigue', 'vicarious trauma' and 'secondary trauma' are often used interchangeably but are not the same. Understanding the differences between these is important in helping you identify the factors that contribute to developing them and to ultimately create ways to prevent and treat them.

Compassion fatigue

Every person who cares about their patient/clients will develop a certain amount of compassion fatigue at some point in their career. If we are engaging empathetically with those whom we support, then we will be impacted by compassion fatigue. It's not something I think we can necessarily avoid. Instead, we implement strategies to prevent tipping the scales into something we find challenging to manage. Compassion fatigue is an occupational hazard and has been described as 'the cost of caring for others in emotional pain'.[1] It is a state of profound mental and physical exhaustion and is often an erosion of our empathy, our compassion and our hope – for others and ourselves.

Consequently, we begin to see changes in our personal and professional lives. For example, we may feel more irritated with our loved ones, feeling distant from them, or that supporting them is a chore or another task to do. At work, we may begin to become intolerant of those we work with and support, contributing to toxic working environments, cynicism or the violation of boundaries. It might be more subtle than this; we might be behaving in the right way, but in our heads we are thinking, 'I've seen or heard much worse.'

A psychotherapist's experience of compassion fatigue

It has been quite full-on at work for the past few months, supporting clients impacted by trauma. I work three days per week and consider myself pretty good at self-care. One evening when I got home from work, the kids were bickering, my husband was asking me something, and I could feel the swell of irritation inside me. I couldn't take it, and I exploded at them all. I looked at their shocked faces and left crying. Later that evening, my husband came to find me, and we talked.

I was physically and emotionally exhausted, and it was increasing. When I was around my family and friends, I felt like I had little space for them emotionally. On reflection, I found it hard to support them when they wanted to talk something through with me or listen. I felt like I had used my empathy, understanding and listening all day at work that I had nothing left to give to those I loved. I felt utterly overloaded.

Some signs that you might be experiencing compassion fatigue are:

- If your empathy, compassion and hope for others and yourself is eroding.
- Personal life: feeling more irritated with your loved ones, feeling distant from them.
- Professional life: increasingly intolerant of your colleagues, becoming cynical, contributing to toxic work environments, violating boundaries.
- Subtle signs: behaving in the right way but thinking, 'I've seen or heard much worse.'

Burnout

Burnout is different from compassion fatigue. Although it can also be characterized by physical and emotional exhaustion, it refers to 'the chronicity, acuity, and complexity that is perceived to be beyond the capacity of the service provider'. Usually, feelings of burnout emerge over time gradually. People describe that their drive, enthusiasm and motivation have diminished, and they feel worn out. Many people can identify direct stressors, either in work or their personal life, that contribute to it, and when these are no longer there, or they change job, the feelings resolve.

In 2019, the World Health Organization (WHO) revised the 11th edition of the *International Classification of Diseases* to recognize burnout as an occupational phenomenon instead of a medical condition. This shift acknowledges that burnout syndrome results from chronic workplace stress,[2] highlighting the need for organizations to create working environments that optimize mental wellbeing.

Working in the helping profession makes us more vulnerable to burnout due to gruelling rotas, low pay, lack of resources, and demanding work environments. It can be experienced alongside compassion fatigue or vicarious trauma and affect any profession. Many believe there is currently a burnout syndrome epidemic affecting those working in healthcare.[3]

Some signs that you might be experiencing burnout are:

- reduced drive, enthusiasm and motivation
- feeling physically, emotionally and psychologically worn out.

Moral suffering

When someone feels powerless to carry out the ethical decision they deem as appropriate that can create feelings of moral distress. When this distress is experienced repeatedly with long term consequences this can be deemed moral injury. Moral suffering is a much broader term to encompass both of these.

Moral distress has been described as being pervasive among helping professionals. It has been defined as something that occurs as a 'decision that needs to be made without being able to make it, usually as a result of various hurdles: institution policy, lack of time, protocol'.[4] Essentially, having to make decisions that we fundamentally disagree with or are morally opposed to can lead to deeply held feelings of powerlessness, shame, guilt, compassion fatigue, and symptoms of post-traumatic stress disorder (PTSD).

Moral injury has been described as a traumatic event or events that includes perpetrating, failing to prevent, or bearing witness to actions that 'transgress deeply held moral beliefs and expectations'.[5] Like moral distress, those with moral injury may experience shame, frustration and guilt. In practice, I often see workers who experience moral distress or injury as their spirits being broken and a profound sense of shame. Although neither is a mental illness, moral injury is often a precursor to PTSD. Below are a range of examples from staff impacted by moral distress and injury.

Some examples of potential moral injurious events are:[6]

- having to choose which of two equally unwell patients is provided with specific care;
- where colleagues or patients are put in danger because of your indecision or lack of experience;
- failure to report serious clinical incidents, near misses, or bullying of yourself, colleagues or patients;
- witnessing or contributing to a decision made, or not made, that resulted in the harm or death of patients.

Junior doctor

I was four hours into my 12-hour shift, having worked a string of seven shifts. I was paged to assist, as a patient had gone into cardiac arrest. When I arrived on the ward, one of the nursing staff informed me that the patient had a DNR ('Do Not Resuscitate') but that the family members had overridden it. Some staff had already begun life-saving measures, and I started assisting them. Our efforts were in vain, and the patient died. However, it left me with a deep sense of embarrassment and guilt. I didn't feel able to intervene, ask my colleagues to stop, respect the DNR, and speak with the family. I felt shame that I had gone against what the patient had wanted and that we had used resources and time unnecessarily.

Social worker

Having worked in addiction services for over 20 years, I've seen my share of cases, and over that time, our caseloads have become overwhelming to manage. One case which particularly stands out is with a young service user, where we had fought hard to get funding for them to go into a drug rehabilitation unit. He had been funded for the full 12-week programme. After successfully completing this, there was an option for him to attend a day unit for further support, and the team felt he would do well here. However, I received contact from the unit to say they had discharged him after the 12 weeks, and his place wasn't funded for the day programme.

Due to the volume of my workload, I had forgotten to submit the paperwork for funding. By the time I had done this, and his place was approved, he had returned to using drugs, had overdosed, and sadly died. Even now, I am plagued by 'what if's', and the notion of self-forgiveness is a distant one. I don't feel I deserve forgiveness.

Intensivist

Working in the Intensive Care Unit during COVID-19, we had limited beds and equipment. Decision-making was shared between the staff as to how best to treat patients. We couldn't treat everyone, and there just weren't enough resources. I know people would probably have survived if there were, and even though it isn't directly my fault, I can't help feeling responsible. I came into medicine to save lives, and I haven't. I don't know how I feel about that.

Midwife

I still feel haunted by that day. Being involved in a baby's death goes entirely against what I came into this profession to do. And yet, I missed the signs. I was tired, we were seriously short-staffed, and I didn't listen to the mum when she shared her concerns with me. I didn't have time. I wept with the family when I passed them their baby. At that moment, I knew that I had a part to play in their baby's death. I was deeply sorry, and I said so.[7]

Signs that you might be experiencing moral distress/moral injury are feelings of:

- powerlessness
- shame
- guilt
- compassion fatigue
- symptoms of PTSD.

2
Trauma responses

Work-related primary and secondary trauma

Direct trauma is often the result of contact with a persistent, intense event that involves death or the threat of death, injury, or physical safety to you. Traumatic events are defined by these features and don't necessarily mean that you will develop trauma-related symptoms. There are a range of responses experienced as a result of the traumatic events, which might be physically and/or psychologically wounding (trauma distress) for you.

Examples of work-related trauma could be:[1]

- workplace violence
- bullying
- medical errors and complications
- death and serious injury.

With secondary trauma, you are not in direct danger. Instead, you either witness, are told or read about a traumatic event. It could also be, for example, that you are supporting someone who has suffered a severe assault, and they are retelling their experience about what has happened and its impact on them.

Exposure to either primary or secondary trauma can lead to post-traumatic stress disorder (PTSD). This is an anxiety disorder in which the person might experience one or more of the following symptoms after the traumatic event (or series of traumatic events): avoidance behaviours (not wanting to be reminded in any way about the event), re-experiencing (nightmares, flashbacks), or constantly feeling on edge (anxious, difficulty concentrating, anger, irritability). Understandably, it can be a very frightening and potentially isolating time as you try to 'make sense' of your experience.

Vicarious trauma

Vicarious trauma is not a single traumatic exposure event or a series of events. Instead, it is a culmination of hearing, witnessing, or reading about multiple individuals' experiences of trauma. Probably, you won't recall them all, and it is like emotional wounding by a thousand stories. Each one has an impact, and those affected by vicarious trauma find that their beliefs about the world alter, and the images or events they have been exposed to become challenging to forget. We absorb these images and events as if we had experienced them, even though the trauma did not happen to us. This can create feelings of profound sadness, anger at the world, and numbness, and result in our being emotionally overwhelmed. In my experience, vicarious trauma can often be the result of multiple secondary traumatic events.

Child protection administrator's vicarious trauma and compassion fatigue

I have worked in the same service for over 20 years, and I love my work and the team. All case notes are electronic now, but before that, I would have to input some of the case information into the computer. When I first started, I found it really hard reading the things that had happened to these poor kids. It would keep me up at night, and when I had my own children, I had to find a way for it not to affect me. So, I would listen to music while I was doing it or think of something else. It worked, and for quite a few years, I could cope really well with it. Then we were encouraged to move over to electronic case notes exclusively. For the past six months, this involved any new cases needing input onto the new system. For months, I sat at my desk reading hundreds of things that had happened to these children. I just couldn't detach myself from it. I began to have panic attacks before going into work, and I would have images in my head from some of the things I had read. Even though I felt exhausted, I couldn't sleep and was tearful all the time. I didn't know what was happening to me until I spoke with our service manager, and she suggested I talk to someone. This is when I first heard about vicarious trauma.

Signs you might be experiencing primary or secondary trauma:

- avoidance behaviours (not wanting to be reminded in any way about the event);

- re-experiencing (nightmares, flashbacks);
- feeling constantly on edge (anxious, difficulty concentrating, anger, irritability).

Signs you might be experiencing vicarious trauma are feelings of:

- sadness
- anger at the world
- numbness
- being emotionally overwhelmed.

3
Our brain's response to trauma

Many parts of the brain are involved with understanding how the body and brain function during trauma, including the prefrontal cortex (front brain), the limbic system (located in the centre of the brain), and the brain stem (which is located at the base of the brain and controls the flow of messages from the brain to the rest of the body).

During a traumatic experience, adrenaline rushes through the body, and the memory is imprinted into the amygdala, which is part of the limbic system and stores all the emotional significance of the event. However, rather than holding the trauma memory like a story, it reserves sensory fragments, that is, how our five senses were experiencing the trauma as it happened. The memories are stored through elements of tastes, touch, smells, sounds and visual images.

Triggers

Being triggered is more than just emotional discomfort. For many, it can be an extreme emotional response that reminds the individual of a traumatic or emotionally distressing event (a 'trigger'). The autonomic nervous system is comprised of two parts: the sympathetic and the parasympathetic nervous system. The sympathetic nervous system activates the flight/fright/freeze/flop response during a threat or perceived danger, and the parasympathetic system restores the body to a state of calm.

The brain can be easily triggered after trauma by sensory input, and normal circumstances can be perceived as threatening or dangerous. These triggers can be internal (coming from within us) and can be anything from a physical sensation, taste in our mouth, position our body is in, to a memory or emotion. External triggers can be within our environments and could be a person, a place, an object, a smell or a situation. The sensory fragments are misinterpreted, and the brain has difficulty distinguishing between what an actual threat is, and what is non-threatening. Some people feel like they are 'reliving' the event. It is vital to know that it is not happening again. Instead, you are 'recalling' a difficult memory, which understandably might feel emotionally painful and frightening.

During a traumatic event, or when someone is triggered, they enter a fight/flight/freeze/flop state. Due to the trauma, the brain becomes overwhelmed. As the body goes into survival mode, the rational part of their brain (prefrontal cortex) involved in problem-solving, risk assessment, and making meaning of language goes offline.

Our brains are hardwired to make associations, and so even if something has a vague connection with the traumatic event, this could be enough to trigger an emotional response. Most of the information we process is on a subconscious level on any given day, and so your body might respond to a trigger you may not be consciously aware of. When triggered, it does not necessarily mean you are in danger, but your brain is reacting as if you are. Therefore, learning to calm and soothe your mind and body will help your brain learn to decipher between actual and perceived threats.

A paramedic's trauma being triggered

We had a call put through as usual. My adrenaline is always a little bit higher when I know I'm going to an incident with potentially multiple fatalities. When we arrived at the scene, it was like nothing I had ever experienced before, and it was like something from a movie. There was debris everywhere, people running, screaming, there were bodies and body parts all around. I went into autopilot, went out there, and did my job.

A couple of years later, we were doing some renovation work in our house. I was really enjoying it, much more than I thought. One of the days, I was demolishing lots of the internal walls and had just finished. I took my mask and goggles off. At that moment, I inhaled a massive cloud of dust, and I could hardly see for the dust and debris.

I had what I can only describe as a panic attack. The taste of the dust, the vision of debris and dust... I felt like I had been transported back to the scene of that horrific day, and the images that I thought I had buried away came back at that moment.

4

The wonder nerve

As mentioned, in the autonomic nervous system, there are two primary components: the parasympathetic (rest/digest) and sympathetic systems (flight/fright/freeze/flop). There are three pathways within the parasympathetic system which are all working to ensure our survival. These are the dorsal vagal, which is the oldest part of the system and manages organs involved in our digestion. The sympathetic system evolved next, enabling us to mobilize (fight and flight) and support blood circulation, regular heart rhythms, temperature changes, and responses when we have postural changes. The ventral vagal system was the last to be built and is unique to mammals. It allows us to form social connections and communication, and its main job is overseeing the sympathetic and dorsal systems to ensure they work in harmony.

The vagus nerve is a significant part of the parasympathetic system and is the longest, most widely distributed cranial nerve in the body, responsible for the mind–body connection. It is a network of neural pathways, and *vagus* in Latin means wandering, which is very apt as it runs from the brain stem to part of the colon. It has some motor functions (it controls the movement of various muscles and the functions of some glands) and sensory functions (it sends information, including details about smells, tastes, sights and sounds to the brain). If we look at how this bidirectional brain–body connection works more closely, we see that the vagus nerve influences organs below our diaphragm while the ventral vagus influences organs above the diaphragm. So, messages are sent in two directions via the dorsal and ventral vagal pathways. Sensory information goes from the body to the brain, and motor information returns from the brain to the body, making our brain–body connection incredibly strong and bountiful.

Like anything in our body that we want to function optimally, we need to use it regularly, and in the case of the vagus nerve, tone it. We can measure how effective our ventral vagus activity (vagal tone) is through our heart rate variability (HRV). This measures the variation in time between our heartbeats. The higher the HRV is, the higher the vagal tone is, enabling us to adjust to life's stressors and have a flexible autonomic nervous system.[1] So, increasing our vagal tone activates the parasympathetic nervous system, our 'rest digest' state, and having a higher vagal tone means that our body can relax faster after stress. Evidence suggests that the vagus nerve has a role to play in managing anxiety, depression and PTSD.

As for helping professions, many of us are working in continually stressful environments. We might be experiencing heightened levels of distress a lot of the time, which erodes our physical and emotional wellbeing. When our ventral vagal capacity (which helps us feel safe and connected) runs on empty, we move down a step and enter the sympathetic nervous system, so fight/flight experiences are fuelled by adrenalin and cortisol. Now, our system is no longer looking for connections with another; survival is its priority, and complex, flexible reasoning becomes compromised.[2] Connecting with our internal resources and restoring our ventral vagal capacity can be of tremendous help to us.

When I learned about the function of the vagus nerve and how toning it could positively impact mental wellbeing, I was hooked. I try to keep this quote by Hippocrates in my head: 'The natural healing force within each one of us is the greatest force in getting well.' In the chapters that follow, I will suggest ways to learn how to listen to what your autonomic nervous system is telling you and how to tone your vagus nerve to enable you to feel calmer when stressed or distressed.

5

Prevalence of work-related adversity

Over the decades, there has been increasing interest among researchers in defining burnout, compassion fatigue and secondary and vicarious trauma and in understanding the causes and impact of these issues, as well as in investigating their prevention and treatment. There are various opinions on the prevalence of these conditions among the helping professions. Still, there is a consensus that it is a cause for concern and that it is at a crisis level. Not only do these difficulties compromise the mental wellbeing of a workforce, but they result in high levels of absenteeism, have a financial impact on services, compromise patient safety, increase defensive practice, and result in many leaving their profession. Many of us are experiencing and witnessing first-hand the impact of burnout, compassion fatigue and trauma on our colleagues, services, and those we serve to help.

Some evidence has suggested that between 40 and 85 per cent of helping professionals had high levels of compassion fatigue or traumatic symptoms.[1]

Prevalence of compassion fatigue, burnout and psychological trauma in some helping professions

Midwives (UK)

From a study of nearly 2000 midwives, over half experienced burnout due to work and over one-third had high levels of stress, anxiety and depression.[2] This is particularly the case for midwives under the age of 40, having less than ten years of experience, working in a clinical midwifery setting, and having a disability. The emotional wellbeing of UK midwives is worse than that of midwives in other countries.[3]

Clinical social workers (USA)

A study examining the levels of secondary traumatic stress (STS), compassion fatigue, burnout and compassion satisfaction in 256 social workers found that many experienced significant STS levels, and 40 per cent met the criteria for PTSD.[4]

Doctors and medical students (Australia)
The National Mental Health Survey of Doctors and Medical Students,[5] which included a sample of 12,252 doctors, and 1811 medical students, found that doctors reported significantly higher rates of psychological distress and suicidal thoughts than both the general Australian population and other Australian professions.

Child protection workers (Norway)
In a study of 506 child protection workers, 70 per cent reported moderate burnout symptoms, and almost 37 per cent displayed moderate symptoms of secondary trauma.[6]

These examples provide a brief snapshot of compassion fatigue, burnout, PTSD and vicarious and secondary trauma even before the COVID-19 pandemic hit us. We still do not yet know the full impact that the pandemic has had on the mental wellbeing of those working in the helping professions.

However, what is known is that there has been an increase in feelings of anxiety, depression, PTSD, and moral injuries in staff across the world. Evidence suggests that 13 to 26 months after the 2006 SARS outbreak, there was a significant increase in burnout, psychological distress and PTSD[7] among healthcare workers. Before the pandemic, it had been well established that PTSD has associated comorbidities such as alcohol dependence, anxiety, depression, drug misuse and suicide among healthcare workers.[8]

Emerging research has highlighted that many healthcare staff caring for patients who tested positive for COVID-19 reached the threshold for severe depression, PTSD, severe anxiety or problem drinking,[9] with nursing staff more affected than physicians. It could be due to the empathetic nature and caregiver–patient relationship often present in nursing staff.[10]

Within the helping professions, some are potentially at higher risk of developing burnout or trauma. For example, in cross-sectional studies, younger nurses, or those with less experience, have demonstrated higher levels of compassion fatigue and burnout.[11] It could be that the transition from training to working as a qualified nurse involves long working hours and the requirement to develop additional clinical skills in a challenging environment. A study of 15,000 physicians found a ten-point gap in self-reported burnout rates between women and men.[12] It could be that women have more demands on them and are trying to balance personal and family needs, particularly during child-bearing years. The expression of burnout differs, with women physicians suffering from emotional exhaustion, while their male colleagues tend to express depersonalization. It could be that gender-based differences are present due to the manifestation of burnout, for example in emotional exhaustion, making it easier to identify in women.

If you think you might be experiencing any of the above – compassion fatigue, burnout, trauma or stress – or think you might be at risk of developing them, you are by no means alone: many others feel the same way. There are also positive, actionable and manageable steps you can take to improve your mental wellbeing.

Like, I'm sure, many of you reading this book, I have experienced high levels of burnout and compassion fatigue at times throughout my career, and never more so than when I started working in mental health at the age of 22.

My story of burnout and compassion fatigue

My first experience was working as a mental health coordinator at an evening drop-in centre for homeless people. My role was to engage and support service users to attend mainstream mental health and physical health services. So, I would help them during the daytime wherever they were, and in the evening, they would attend the drop-in service. I had never done any work like this before and had not applied therapeutic interventions. However, it was a small team, with weekly supervision with a psychotherapist, daily spaces to 'offload', and weekly wellbeing meetings. I felt very much supported and psychologically safe.

Most of those who attended had suffered horrific childhood traumas, which I found very difficult to listen to at times due to the gruesome and cruel actions inflicted on them by others. While living on the streets, their vulnerabilities, alongside doing what they needed to survive, was sometimes overwhelming for me to listen to. It was a brutal entry into the world of physical and emotional trauma. When I returned home some evenings, I didn't know how to come down from what I had listened to or witnessed that day. Unknowingly at the time, I took on the role of rescuer, and at times my boundaries became blurred. I would sometimes start my shift hours earlier to support someone, or a service user would have allocated me – without consulting me – as their next of kin. I would get a call in the middle of the night, having to go to the hospital as they had usually overdosed on drugs. In every instance, I went.

I became a birth partner for many women who were sex workers, and when they had birthed, their baby was either taken into care, was on medication to help them withdraw from substances, or sadly died. I can still recall so vividly a particular service user who had found out she was pregnant. She had worked so incredibly hard to find and keep her accommodation and remain drug-free during her pregnancy. Her three previous children had been taken into care, and she was determined it wouldn't happen this time. She attended all her antenatal appointments. As her birth partner, I couldn't help but get wrapped in her bubble of joy; such hope we shared – this time, it would be different. I received a phone call during the night to say she had gone into premature labour at six months. As I drove to the hospital, I recalled having left her earlier that day, when she had been happily folding some baby clothes she had bought. I held her and her baby, who died, as she wept. The emotion from her permeated into me, and at that moment, it was as if I could feel her heart breaking. There were no words of comfort to offer. That morning, like any other, the sun rose, and life carried on. I went to work, and the service user returned to the streets and the life she had known.

After that experience, I had a more profound understanding of why it didn't feel like a choice for many to use substances; living with their past pain was unbearable, and numbing that was their only focus.

Months later, I received a phone call informing me that I was next of kin for a service user whom I had been supporting for the past two years, and who was close to death. I sat, not knowing what to do; I was, I think, in shock. He had suffered horrific physical, sexual and psychological abuse for many years of his childhood. His vulnerability was there physically and emotionally when we first met, and we clicked. We shared a similar sense of humour, and we chatted about the big and the small stuff. He was clear he wanted a life of sobriety, to have his own place, and forge something meaningful with his life, and he did. He became sober throughout our working relationship, maintained it, and adjusted to having his own home. As I drove to the hospital that evening, a tsunami of questions flooded my mind: 'What's happened?'; 'Have they got the right person?' But they hadn't been mistaken. When I arrived, there he was. I took a breath, went over to him, took his hand, and told him I was here. He briefly opened his eyes and softly said, 'This is shit, isn't it?' Those were his last words to me.

When he died, I struggled. I was angry at the injustice of his death and overwhelmed with sadness. I was grieving his loss and found it challenging to be present at work or in my personal life.

For nearly five years, I worked in that post, and the decision to leave was not an easy one. I was physically and emotionally exhausted, and I was beginning to have less compassion and empathy for those I supported. I knew it was time to go.

Reflecting on my experiences in that role, I learned the meaning of having boundaries with those I support, the importance of self-care, and how my history impacts the work I do. These were some of the biggest lessons I was gifted so early in my career and ones that I've carried with me throughout.

Working in a helping profession usually involves navigating emotionally intense environments. Some people find comfort knowing others have also experienced something similar to them and relate to their feelings. Often, it can be the first step towards healing. As you navigate your way through this book, I hope you feel inspired to create ways to support your mental wellbeing, to enable you to live the personal and professional life you undoubtedly deserve.

Part I
OPTIMIZING YOUR MENTAL WELLBEING

There is growing popularity to talk about health and social care staff practising self-care. While I wholeheartedly agree with this, I think there is a gaping absence in training our existing teams and students entering the helping profession to look after themselves. Practising self-care is a skill. Many staff are left utterly vulnerable to compromised mental wellbeing and illness at some point in their careers. Helping professions aren't taught ways to look after themselves while navigating systems with limited resources, bullying cultures, staff shortages, low morale, and psychologically unsafe working environments.

Ideally, to reduce the impact of burnout, vicarious trauma and compassion fatigue, changes would be implemented top-down (on an organizational and team level) and bottom-up (on an individual level). This book focuses primarily on providing ways to support staff as individuals. That is not by any means to say it is the sole responsibility of individual staff to manage their own wellbeing and negate the responsibility of organizations and leaders to embed staff wellbeing into their culture. Instead, it is an offering: for those of you out there working in an organization that doesn't value your mental wellbeing, there are ways you can protect yourself. For those working in a system where staff wellbeing is at the heart of the organization, the suggestions outlined are here to inspire you.

The suggestions proposed throughout this book might feel foreign to many of you. They might be things you've never tried before and could be very much out of your comfort zone. Expect this to happen when trying new things, especially if it's for the first time. You deserve to be as psychologically healthy as you can be, for yourself, those you support in your role, and for your family and friends. It all begins with asking yourself how willing you are to make changes that will be long lasting. So, maybe before trying some of the suggestions here, ask yourself:

On a scale of 1–10, how willing am I to feel the discomfort of trying this (0 being *not willing* and 10 being *completely willing*)?

It might be worth reminding yourself of something you initially tried, that you found difficult, and that was uncomfortable, but that you felt better doing it with regular practice. Many of us do everything we can to avoid feeling discomfort. Learning to tolerate our discomfort can support us to strengthen our confidence in overcoming challenges.

This section provides ways to develop new habits and change existing behaviours, addressing how you can after yourself. There are a range of suggestions to encourage you to start thinking about your mental wellbeing and to help you mitigate the impact of burnout, compassion fatigue and trauma during your career, irrespective of where on that journey you are.

6
Building a foundation

New Year's resolutions, diets, exercise regimes, quitting smoking, starting yoga... the list could be endless. How many times have we set a plan or intended to be healthier and take better care of our mental and physical wellbeing, and, for lots of different reasons, haven't been able to maintain it. We might have put a plan in place, and then we have deviated from it, and eventually returned to our old way of being. If this sounds familiar to you, you're not on your own.

There are multimillion-dollar industries devoted to making us believe that, if we look better, smell better, are more successful, work harder, or are thinner, then we will be happier. At that moment, signing up for a subscription, joining a group, or purchasing the latest fad is seductive because it's easy to do; we just have to click a button. Changing our behaviour and habits is tough, however. We are hard-wired for predictability, and so when we have a routine that we feel secure in, it takes lots of motivation to behave differently. I think that making suggestions about ways to look after our wellbeing is redundant in the absence of knowing how to change our behaviour and create new habits.

Helping professions understand the need to have protected breaks, eat and drink while on shift, and manage their stress levels. We know that knowledge alone is not enough to change our behaviour; other ingredients are required, too. Evidence suggests that for the desired behaviour (B) to occur, an interaction between three necessary conditions is required: Capability (C), Opportunity (O) and Motivation (M).[1] For example, to optimize mental wellbeing (B), we must be physically and psychologically able to do so at any given time (C). We then need to have the physical and social opportunity (O) to do the behaviour; and, at that moment, want/need to do the behaviour more than any other competing behaviours, that is, to be sufficiently motivated (M). Motivation includes automatic processes (habits/impulses) and reflective processes (intention/choice).

Strengthening our motivation in order to engage in the desired behaviour is required, for example, by developing appropriate beliefs and reducing the motivation to continue with the undesired behaviour. Maximizing our ability to manage emotions by developing relevant skills and specific plans to change will help enhance supportive activities, for example eliciting social support and changing routines/environment. Researchers at Duke University (Durham, North Carolina) have reported that habits account for 40 per cent of our behaviours each day.[2] So, learning ways to create different habits to improve our likelihood of following new ones that support our mental wellbeing is useful.

When changing our behaviour, many of us have 'good' intentions; we intend to go to the gym after work, so we pack our gym bag and plan when we might go. But then, when it comes to going, we don't quite make it there, for countless reasons. When this happens, we've just fallen into what's known as the intention–behaviour gap. Evidence suggests that this happens due to habits, hedonic goals (focusing on improving feelings in a particular situation), or impulses automatically influencing our behaviour. The good news is there are many strategies we can put in place to increase our success in avoiding the intention–behaviour gap.

Goal setting

It is not enough to change our behaviour by just setting a goal. We need to create the right conditions to support us to be able to achieve what we have developed. Research indicates that positively framed approach goals are more supportive in helping us move towards the outcomes we want, whereas avoidance goals do the opposite and move us away from where we want to be.[3,4] For example, a positively framed approach goal might be 'When I am at work today, I will have my break and eat some food,' compared with a negatively framed avoidance goal like 'I'm not going to miss my lunch break today.'

Despite both of these approaches appearing to promote protecting your lunch break, there are different emotional and cognitive processes involved. Positive emotions, thoughts and greater psychological wellbeing are associated with approach goals, whereas higher negative feelings and fewer positive thoughts are linked to avoidance goals. Therefore, setting approach goals will help us learn ways to integrate strategies to protect ourselves emotionally.

Knowing why we want to make the changes is essential, as this can support us with our motivation. Significant changes can happen over time if we:

- set small, achievable goals which feel easy;
- specify when and where we will do it, preferably tagging it onto an existing habit;
- practise every day, which can be tagged onto existing habits.

Below I've used the example of pursuing the goal of mindful breathing as an illustration.

Example of goal setting

What is my overall goal?
Practise mindfulness for five minutes daily.

Why is it important for me to pursue this goal?
I want to feel calmer and more present in my work and personal life to be the nurse and mum I want to be.

When will I start my goal?
Monday 14th at 6:30 am.

When will I practice it?
When making a hot drink in the morning between 6:30 am and 7 am.

Day 1: While waiting for the hot water to boil for my coffee, I will practise 30 seconds of mindful breathing.

Day 2: While waiting for the hot water to boil for my coffee, I will practise 40 seconds of mindful breathing.

Day 3: While waiting for the hot water to boil for my coffee, I will practise 50 seconds of mindful breathing.

Day 4: While waiting for the hot water to boil for my coffee, I will practise 60 seconds of mindful breathing.

By continuing this pattern, adding ten seconds each day means that I am creating consistency, and in 30 days, I would be practising five minutes of mindful breathing each day. Integrating the new habit alongside an existing one (e.g. making a coffee) will help it feel more manageable and more likely to be remembered. In the beginning, when incrementally increasing it, if it's feeling tough, break it down into smaller, bitesize chunks. We might not consistently achieve what we hoped for each day, so if you miss one day, try not to miss two days of practice in a row.

What if?

Often, we will begin to try new things when our motivation is high, and we feel determined to make a change. However, for various reasons, over time, our motivation wavers, and factors in our environment mean we struggle to continue pursuing our goal with the same ferocity we once did. Identifying what these barriers might be in advance of starting to change our behaviour can support us in maintaining any changes. It is more likely that we will revert to old habits if we haven't set up the necessary environment to help them succeed.

Barriers can be both internal and external. Internal barriers might be thoughts, feelings and experiences that we find difficult to manage or tolerate. They can impact on our motivation and potentially sabotage our new habits from succeeding.

External barriers could be anything in our environment, work or relationships. Our brains are highly tuned to making links between situations, our environment and how we feel. For example, my morning routine involves having a coffee when I come downstairs. I don't even think about it. I mindlessly will perform all of the actions because my brain has associated morning time with coffee. Therefore, the situational/environmental cue (kitchen, morning time) means that my brain knows what to do because I have repeated this action daily. It is positively reinforced (I feel good when I have the coffee). Repetition and reinforcement are vital components in habit formation. Conversely, we increase the likelihood of forming new habits when they are tagged onto existing ones.

Willpower ebbs and flows throughout the day, and yet many of us feel like our willpower dictates whether we are motivated to pursue our goal and stick at it. This isn't the case: If–Then planning[5] can support us in our goal pursuit. These are self-made plans which require us to do a particular thing in a specific situation, and because they are pre-specified, this tends to reduce the reliance on our willpower.

If–Then plans have shown to be a highly effective strategy, increasing our chances of reaching our goal by up to 300 per cent by helping us form our desired habits.

There are two steps to creating If–Then plans. I will stay with the example of pursuing the goal to practise five minutes of mindful breathing.

- Step 1 (If): Identify situations when I'm unlikely to practise mindful breathing.
- Step 2 (Then): Create ways to overcome these.

Step 1 (If): Situations	Step 2 (Then): Solutions
If I am in a rush in the morning and don't have time	Then I will set a reminder on my phone to do it later when I return home and ensure I leave enough time in the morning to practise
If I'm feeling too tired and don't feel motivated to do it	Then I will remind myself why it is important to me to pursue this goal
If I forget to practise	Then I will set a reminder on my phone that will prompt me the night before, or I will leave a note beside the coffee pot
If I have a lot on my mind and don't feel able to try it	Then I will make a smaller goal of practice for that day

Remember, we are hard-wired for an association, and If–Then planning is successful because the situation and the action become linked in our mind. Our brain recognizes the situation as an opportunity to advance goal achievement, and so when it is detected, it automatically initiates the actions. An additional benefit to If–Then planning is that it also builds self-talk, which we will explore later in the book.

Support network

There are many different forms of support, and thinking about what we might need to increase the likelihood of achieving our goals is useful. If we need more information about doing something (e.g. meditation), we might enrol in a group, workshop or course. Also, practically, there might be things that need to be in place to incorporate new habits into our daily lives.

For many of us, sharing our goals with those in our support network (friends, spouse, family) can help us in our pursuit of achieving our goals. Often, our support network provides us with emotional support, championing us and providing encouragement when we might need it the most. Some evidence suggests that sharing our goals, and our weekly progress, with a friend can increase the success of achieving and maintaining the change because, socially, it holds us to account.[6] Accountability and public commitment can act as drivers in our goal pursuit, which sharing with a friend or friends serves.

Feeling that we have others around us who are supportive can provide us with a sense of security and increase our feelings of self-worth. Identifying who in our life will be the person/people who will positively support our goals could help us successfully achieve them.

Is it working?

When we're putting effort into creating new habits, we like to see results. It's an indicator that it's working and that our hard work hasn't been in vain. This requires us to monitor our progress and review it, and to be open-minded to changing our approach if needed.

Often, our more destructive habits, like smoking cigarettes, drug use or excessive alcohol intake, are quickly formed because using them activates the reward system in our brain (through the dopamine transmitter). So, even though we might not want to do it, we're naturally rewarded, which continues usage. However, with other positive habits like mindfulness, exercise and healthy eating, although through consistent practice they eventually activate our reward system, this doesn't happen straight away, as in substance use. Therefore, when starting out, our reward system might need some help. We can do this by setting rewards, for example: 'After week one of practising mindful breathing, I plan to sit outside in nature for five minutes on my own.'

During the pandemic, we all had to rethink how we live our lives, connect with others, socialize, school our children, and work. Adam Grant is an organizational psychologist at Wharton University. In his book *Think Again: The Power of Know What You Don't Know*, he writes about how we should try to think like scientists. According to Grant, this means treating our strategy as a hypothesis and our product as an experiment. So, in the case of forming new habits to optimize our wellbeing: we set our goal, we think through the factors which may or may not help us achieve it (hypothesis), we practise doing it (experiment), then review it, and make adjustments if needed by thinking about why it may or may not be working (rethinking).

The template below is a guide to helping you begin to create new habits to support your mental wellbeing. If you're not sure what your goal is, that's okay. It might be that you will complete this exercise once you have read through the book and have a clearer idea of ways to optimize your wellbeing.

Exercise

Creating new habits

What is my goal?

Why is it important for me to pursue this goal?

When will I start my goal?

When will I practise it?

What needs to be in place before I begin pursuing my goal?

Barriers

Internal (thoughts, feelings, etc.)	External (environment, situational)

If–Then Plan

Step 1 (If): Situations	Step 2 (Then): Solutions

Which supportive person(s) can I share my goal with?

What are the signs to me I am benefitting from this goal?

How will I reward myself when I have reached it?

What date will I review how effective it is?

What changes (if any) do I need to make?

7

Our emotional language

Emotions are one of the biggest things that make us humans, yet we constantly receive the message that we should be happy and think positive, as though all the other feelings are less relevant. As humans, our emotions are complex; they can be messy, uncomfortable, inconvenient and challenging to navigate. Who wants to feel vulnerable? It can be an exposing and lonely place to be. Yet, I've never heard anyone share with me that they regretted it when they went through the tough times, experienced a range of feelings, and came out the other side. Was it hard? Absolutely. Was it painful? Yes. But they share that their quality of life is richer for it. So, there's something about not just going *through* the process but *connecting* with it.

Denying how we feel means we are turning our back on ourselves; we are saying our feelings don't deserve to be seen, we're not worthy of healing or showing kindness to ourselves. We're also short-changing those around us because we avoid connection with another person by denying or suppressing how we feel. These beliefs we hold about experiencing and expressing emotions might have been passed down to us by other people or picked up somewhere along the way. So, they mightn't even belong to us. It could be that over time, while we've been working in the helping profession, that our emotions have slowly eroded. We don't connect with ourselves anymore; we are numb and disconnected.

Research has shown that most of us cannot identify the causes of our emotions and how to manage them. Since 2006, research professor Brené Brown and her team have carried out research asking individuals to write down names of the feelings they can recognize in themselves and others. Consistently, there are only three emotions that people recognize: feeling bad, sad and glad.

Many of the activities in this book are to support your mental wellbeing. They rely on you turning *towards* yourself, connecting with how you feel in your body, and label what this is. However, not everyone has been taught the language of feelings, which makes it difficult to express them so that others might understand.

In my experience, for those whose feelings language is absent or not as developed, often more nuanced emotions get swept into a giant umbrella feeling term. For example, feeling annoyed or frustrated is shared as anger; feeling tearful or disappointed is identified as sad. Being able to label our emotions and share them with another forges a connection. It opens the possibility of understanding why we might be feeling as we do and how we might work through it. Some examples of what broader emotions represent are shared below:

- **Anger** is often about a perceived injustice.
- **Happiness** is a high-energy emotion usually linked to the success of something.
- **Disappointment** is often about our expectations being unmet.
- **Anxiety** is feeling unease, mainly when the outcome is uncertain.
- **Guilt** is feeling psychologically uncomfortable about something we've done or failed to do.
- **Shame** is an intensely painful feeling that we are flawed in some way.

Susan David is a psychologist at Harvard Medical School, an emotions researcher, and author of *Emotional Agility: Get Unstuck, Embrace Change and Thrive in Work and Life*. There she provides some umbrella terms for feelings and then other emotions the broader term might represent:

Sad	Angry	Anxious	Embarrassed
Disappointed	Irritated	Afraid	Lonely
Mournful	Annoyed	Confused	Inferior
Depress	Offended	Stressed	Pathetic
Regretful	Spiteful	Vulnerable	Ashamed
Disillusioned	Frustrated	Sceptical	Guilty
Pessimistic	Grumpy	Worried	Confused
Tearful	Defensive	Cautious	Self-conscious
Dismayed	Disgusted	Nervous	Isolated

Happy		Hurt	
Thankful		Jealous	
Content		Isolated	
Trusting		Betrayed	
Comfortable		Shocked	
Excited		Victimized	
Relieved		Tormented	
Elated		Deprived	
Confident		Abandoned	

Exercise: Defining your emotions

Take a recent situation where you experienced a strong emotion and try to connect with the feelings you felt at the time.

What were the broader emotions you were feeling (hurt, sadness, happiness, anger)?

_____

_____

Now, try to connect with the emotion that might be under that? (You can use the table above as a prompt to help you.)

_____

_____

_____

8
Who are you?

This isn't a fluffy question about your favourite colour, music or food. Instead, it's something much more profound: discovering who you are as a person and how that impacts the work you do. It is a journey to get to know the parts of yourself hidden, buried deep, or that lie quiet, dormant. Getting to know yourself is by no means for the faint-hearted. To connect with your failings, vulnerabilities, prejudices, discriminations and insecurities takes a tremendous amount of courage. Given the challenges you might face while on this journey, it is advisable that no one coerces or manipulates you to do it. Instead, it might be born from a need or desire to change in some way.

There are many benefits to having greater knowledge about who we are. Here are some examples:

- **Greater fulfilment:** knowing what we want and expressing it to those around us can help us feel less frustrated and better understood.
- **Understanding others:** when we connect with our misgivings and struggles, it can help us empathize with others.
- **Being genuine:** when our behaviours match our feelings and values, we often experience less internal conflict.
- **Greater control:** being connected to how we feel and our triggers means that we are better prepared to implement ways to help us feel emotionally safe when needed.

An integral part of working in health and social care is connecting with others and building relationships. Sometimes, building rapport and trust with those in our care needs to be done relatively quickly. For example, if a patient comes into the emergency department requiring lifesaving treatment and they are highly distressed, at that moment, alongside medical interventions, helping them to feel calm will also be vital. Not being able to connect with ourselves potentially stifles our ability to communicate with others.

We seldom talk about our own psychological and emotional vulnerability working in the health and social care sector. Most of us are immersed in a culture that influences and moulds our beliefs and behaviours, and we are rarely prepared and taught how to recognize and manage its impact. It is not uncommon to safeguard ourselves from this vulnerability, and often create a suit of armour made up of professional expertise and sometimes status. Quite rightly so, because we can't save every patient, care does not always go as expected, and we can't always support clients or service users in the way we would like to. This can cause significant emotional wounding and is a source of potential emotional vulnerability.

However, it is an illusion that we are somehow protected against experiencing it by not connecting with this emotional vulnerability. By denying how we feel, we turn away from ourselves and what we need at some of the most challenging times in our work. This doesn't just hurt us, but it hurts those we are trying to support and help in our roles.

For years, I had such a problematic relationship with my vulnerability because it felt exposing. In part, I think I struggled with it because I didn't fully know what to do with it. I was fine holding the vulnerability of others. It felt more comfortable doing that, but I couldn't do that for myself. Until, that is, I learned it wasn't about self-disclosure or exposing myself unsafely; it was about taking a risk when I didn't always know what the outcome was going to be. It was accepting that being human is to be vulnerable, and *how* we respond to this changes our expectations and relationships with vulnerability. When I sit with a client for the first time and observe how much it has taken for them to make that first appointment or the leader who shares with me that they gathered their team together to ask for critical feedback on a project, *courage* is what I witness.

Exercise: What does vulnerability mean to you?

Many of us have a complicated relationship with the word 'vulnerable', so let's start by thinking about what it means to you.

Write down all the words that come to mind when you think of the word 'vulnerable'.

_____

_____

_____

This exercise is adapted from Brené Brown's work in *Daring Greatly*. Think of **three** examples where you recently felt vulnerable, then answer the following questions for each one

Name the situation – for example, *in work.*

_____

_____

_____

What was the circumstance or trigger? *I couldn't input something into the computer system.*

_____

_____

_____

How did you feel? *I felt stupid and incompetent.*

_____

_____

_____

How might you react if you were daring greatly (i.e., using courage and willingness to engage with those around you)? *Admit I don't know how to do it and ask a colleague for help.*

_____

_____

Body connection

We live in our bodies, and many signs of stress, anxiety, depression, or trauma are symptoms of the body. It's easy to get caught up in thinking that these are healed only by working with emotions and thought patterns. We know the catastrophic health consequences that burnout, trauma, grief and anxiety can have on us. We feel feelings in our body, not in our head, so it is our body that is suffering also. Many have shared their desire to live fully in their experiences, to feel 'alive' in their bodies. Our bodies can't be healed by the mind alone.

Connecting with our body is essential as it is our guide to telling us when we are being triggered, relaxed, tense, anxious, destabilized. I would like to invite you to consider the following to help you connect with how you feel in your body.

Exercise: Connecting how you feel in your body

- Take a moment, breathe in deeply, and exhale fully.
- **How** is my body feeling right now?

_____

_____

- **Where** in my body am I feeling _____?
- **What** is the feeling I am experiencing?

_____

_____

> - If this (area of my body) could speak right now, what would it say?
>
> _____
>
> _____
>
> - Take a moment, breathe in deeply, and exhale fully.

This does not need to be a prolonged exercise. It could be something that you practise throughout your working day when you have a moment or integrate it into part of a practice you already do.

We all have a past and history that might predispose us to experience certain work situations in a way that leaves us feeling overwhelmed or distressed. Many of us think we are in our chosen profession because it is a vocation, a calling. Others have a trauma history and want to make a positive difference. We bring our whole selves to work, despite receiving the message to 'leave our personal lives at the door'.

Experience of being triggered at work

Clinic started in the usual way, busy, rushed, and the waiting room filling up with women. I like the 'buzz' of clinic, everyone knows what they need to do, and we all pull together to get on with it, like a well-oiled machine. I was on to my fifth appointment of the day, congratulating a couple on their long-awaited pregnancy news. I watched tears of joy fall down their cheeks and the tender look they shared between one another. My smile was fixed; I said and did all the right things.

What they couldn't see, nor should they, was that, inside, my heart wasn't just breaking, it was shattered into a million pieces. The week before, I had been the patient who sat on the other side of the consultant's table. My husband and I had shared tears of complete devastation and heartache that we would never have any children of our own.

I knew how to be what I needed to be at work. What I hadn't learned at that time was how I needed to protect my own heart when the very job I loved triggered my own fertility trauma.[1]

Knowing how our history might potentially impact the work we do is essential. If we are not aware of and have healed from these past wounds, it makes us more vulnerable to developing vicarious trauma or being triggered during our working day. The accumulation of this over time will undoubtedly impact on our levels of compassion fatigue and burnout.

Grounding

When we start thinking of something stressful, our amygdala kicks into action. This is the emotional response centre of our brain and helps us prepare for emergency events. However, it is also activated and acts as *if* there is an actual threat when there isn't really. So, thinking something terrible is about to happen will trigger it into action, causing changes in our body to occur such as breathing faster, rapid heartbeat and sweaty palms. The amygdala then interprets these changes in our body as further evidence that something is wrong, activating it again, and so a vicious cycle is created. We become more anxious, and emotionally and physically overwhelmed.

When we are in this cycle, our thoughts might catapult us to an experience or tell us how our future might be, so we aren't in the present moment. Coming back to the present moment helps us to ground and say to that part of our brain, 'Right here, right now, I am safe. There is no danger.' This could be a mantra to say to ourselves in the moment. Our mind convinces us, particularly at times of distress, that certain thoughts are true when they are not. Thoughts are not facts, but, at times, they can be too loud and overwhelming for us to tolerate.

Our minds persuade us that the words they churn out are real. We can learn to observe our thoughts. For example, if my mind is telling me, 'Jan, when you go into work tomorrow and share your idea with the team, everyone will think it's stupid,' I might then start feeling anxious and want to avoid feeling stupid and judged by others. Therefore, I don't take the risk and speak out during a meeting. So, we need to learn to do something different:

- Take a moment.
- Ask yourself – if someone came up to me right now and said what my mind has just said, how would I respond? *I might be a bit shocked, and I might be curious why they're saying that and even challenge it in some way.*

It's unlikely that I would completely accept the stranger's opinion and wholeheartedly agree, yet this is what we tend to do when our minds say things like this to us, mainly when it makes us feel anxious or worried. So, here are a couple of myths about what our minds can do. We can't...

- **predict the future:** look out for thoughts like 'This will happen when/if...'
- **read other people's minds:** look out for thoughts like 'This person will think _____ if I do/say that.'

Thoughts and feelings pass and change, even the difficult ones. So, another mantra might be 'This will pass.'

Grounding techniques are one way to help break the vicious stress cycle, enabling us to refocus on our body in the moment and divert our mind away from stressful or complicated thoughts. When we are connected with how our body feels, we can detect when we might begin to start feeling like this. It might help you to practise these techniques when you initially start to feel tension, stress or anxiety, rather than waiting until you feel overwhelmed or panicked. This will help you to access them more easily when you need them the most.

Exercises: Grounding techniques

The 5-4-3-2-1 grounding technique

This technique uses all five senses to support you to try to get back to the present moment. You can do this sitting down or standing up.

- Take a couple of deep breaths, breathing in fully and out fully. Look around you and aloud, or in your mind, name:

  five things you can see in the room you're in or outside the window

  four things you can feel – it could be the texture of your clothing, an object in front of you, a slight breeze on your skin...

  three things you can hear (birds outside, ticking of your clock, traffic, people talking)

  two things you can smell

  one thing you can taste.

- Finally, a couple of deep breaths, breathing in fully and out fully.

Colour

- Choose a colour, any colour; it doesn't matter.
- How many different shades of that colour can you see in the room you are in or out of the window?
- Choose another colour, and repeat until you notice your feelings beginning to ease.

Counting

Start at 100, and count backwards by 6. This usually requires a lot of concentration.

Others

- Listen to your favourite music.
- Go for a walk.
- Move your body: stretching, dancing, running up and down stairs. Due to the adrenalin pumping through our bodies when we are in this cycle, some people find movement helps displace some of this energy. They are then better prepared to do more calming grounding techniques.

9
Values

Acceptance and commitment therapy (ACT) is a psychotherapeutic approach that uses acceptance and mindfulness, focusing on committed, values-based action to help people change their lives.

When people can connect with their values, they feel more confident and fulfilled in their life. There is a groundswell of evidence demonstrating its efficacy across various issues, including chronic pain, anger, addiction, depression, anxiety and PTSD. There is a growing evidence base of its utility in the workplace, supporting staff's performance and mental wellbeing. I was drawn to ACT because of its versatility and a personal drive to lead a more valued life and use it in my work as a psychologist and coach.

Defining our values

Values can be described as our chosen compass in life. They are the things that we want to stand up for, give us a sense of purpose, and help us be the person we want to be. Values are personally chosen, individual to everyone, and they provide us with a tool to help navigate through life. There is no such thing as having 'correct' values.

They're different from goals. Goals are concrete, achievable events, situations or objects that can be completed, finished or ticked off the list. Goals are not the same as values. For example, if you want to be a caring, attentive and patient nurse, that is a value, an ongoing process. You wouldn't start your next shift and not try to be a caring, attentive and patient nurse because then you would no longer be living that value. In contrast, if you wanted to become a manager, that's a goal – it can be achieved. Once you've got the job, you're the manager.

People value several areas in their lives: family relationships; career or employment; parenting; friendship; health and wellbeing; education; spirituality; recreation; intimate relationships and community. Some values might overlap with one another. For example, if you value yoga practice, that might come under spirituality, recreation, health and wellbeing.

To help you to begin to think about your work-related values, I would invite you to consider the following questions:

- Why did you want to become a _____?
- What do you value in your work?

  _____

  _____

- What kind of worker would you like to be?

  _____

  _____

- If you were living up to your ideal standards, what personal qualities would you like to bring to your work?

  _____

  _____

Exercise: Creating your work-related values

- Write a sentence to summarize your valued direction. For example, *I want to be a caring, attentive and patient nurse.*

  _____

- Rate out of 10 how important this value is to you – where 0 = *low importance* and 10 = *high importance.*

  Low 0 1 2 3 4 5 6 7 8 9 10 High

- Rate how successfully you have lived this value during the past month on a scale of 0 (*not at all successfully*) to 10 (*very successfully*).

Not at all 0 1 2 3 4 5 6 7 8 9 10 Very

- What behaviours might reflect this is your value, for example acts of kindness to patients and colleagues (the more you can list, the better).

_____

_____

_____

Barriers are inevitable, and considering these in advance can help you to think about ways to overcome them when they arise. What might get in the way of you demonstrating this value? Write one or two words to remind you of the barriers you will face to pursue your valued path and strategies to help you accept them.

Barriers	Strategies
Feeling stressed	Take a moment – breathe. Do the 5-4-3-2-1 grounding technique. Tell myself: 'This will pass.'

If we valued a single thing, life might be a little simpler. However, it might not be as rich, complete or dynamic. You can use this same template to think about and define the other values you have in your life.

We can't live a valued life 100 per cent of the time. Defining our values is the more straightforward part of the process. We then have to 'walk the walk'. When our thoughts become loud, and we have tough feelings, sensations or memories, taking valued action might feel challenging. So, observing our thoughts and tolerating our inner world is something we learn to do; it doesn't just happen. We might think that we value something, and it isn't until this value is tested that we realize that we don't. Also, the behaviours that we demonstrate in pursuit of those values will come into conflict with one another, and when this happens, we are faced with thinking that we need to choose which value to pursue at that moment.

Responding to values when goals are conflicted

When something is important to us, and we care about it, we might expect that when behaving in ways that reflect this, we feel good. Although that might be the case, it shouldn't be the expectation. Acting on values will likely bring up painful and difficult feelings *because* we care. The presence of emotional pain might even be an indicator that we are in touch with our values. If we didn't care, it wouldn't affect us emotionally.

Values are not morals or ethics. However, I often see that staff are deeply wounded because their professional values have been conflicted or compromised following a morally injurious event.

Most of us enter the helping profession to provide the best possible care and support, irrespective of a patient's condition, gender, age, sexuality or background. This is often our professional values and moral code. However, working in a system that has pulled us in too many directions, where resources are limited, and where there are staff shortages and constrained budgets have taken their toll. Consequently, we cannot provide the level of care and support we have been trained to deliver. Therefore, we still have the work-related values, but the organization we are working in means we aren't able to act in accordance with these, leaving us feeling compromised, and our moral codes shattered. Fostering self-compassion for the thoughts and feelings relating to their experiences can be helpful to heal from these.

10

Fostering self-compassion

Evidence on the efficacy of practising self-compassion has consistently demonstrated that it predicts lower levels of depression and anxiety.[1] Additionally, individuals with a higher degree of self-compassion have lower amounts of the stress hormone (cortisol) in their bodies.[2] When experiencing higher levels of stress, they are better able to self-soothe and regain emotional control. Therefore, practising self-compassion can be advantageous for those workers in the helping profession.

In the Introduction, we explored the negative impact of compassion fatigue and burnout in the helping professions and those the professionals support and care for. Having self-compassion is one way for us to be more robust against emotional exhaustion and burnout. Learning to be sensitive, respectful and non-judgemental towards ourselves helps us to be sensitive, respectful and non-judgemental towards others.[3] So, by meeting our own needs with empathy and understanding, we are better able to meet others' needs.

There is often a misperception that compassion is learning to be kind to ourselves and others. This is no bad thing, and there are numerous benefits in cultivating kindness, like connectivity with others. However, it is much more than this: Paul Gilbert, a pioneer in the field of compassion research, defines it as 'a basic kindness, with a deep awareness of the suffering of oneself and others'.[4] Valuing our wellbeing can make us feel more courageous to turn into suffering rather than disconnect or turn away from it. Having higher self-compassion levels means we will try to prevent and lessen our suffering rather than be reactive to negative feelings.

Dr Kristin Neff is one of the world's leading experts on self-compassion and states that it comprises three separate constructs: self-kindness, common humanity and mindfulness.

Self-kindness

Applying self-kindness is about showing kindness and under-standing to ourselves when we are hurt or failing at something.[5] Our minds tend to be critical and fall into judgement, which can create difficult feelings for us. Recognizing the impact of this on ourselves and treating ourselves with patience and warmth is showing self-kindness.[6] It takes a significant amount of practice to try to have a different relationship with ourselves.

Exercise: When are you judgemental?

To have greater insight into when your mind might be more critical and judgemental, write down the times you notice this happening and how you respond.

Events, situations or circumstances when I feel critical:
for example, *when I have made a mistake at work.*

_____

What does my mind say?
You're foolish for doing that – can't you get anything right?

_____

How I could respond with patience and kindness?
I was in a rush, I'm tired, and I was trying my best. Next time, I need to give myself a little more time.

_____

It is unrealistic to expect that everything we try to achieve will be successful or that we will do it well. There are many different reasons behind this: it might be that we are not as skilled or experienced in this area: our personality is less suited to what we are trying to do: there are limited resources, or we need support. Therefore, during tough times, treating our worth as uncondi-tional even when we might fall short of our expectations, whether through our thoughts or behaviours, are acts of self-kindness.[7]

Common humanity

COVID-19 has significantly impacted on and continues to impact on the mental health of helping professionals across the world. During this time, many mechanisms supported and optimized the wellbeing of helping professionals, one of which was feeling they were part of something bigger than themselves. Many teams and organizations worked incredibly hard to create a feeling of 'being in it together'. Embedding this into the working culture involved fostering a belief that the difficulties experienced by staff are a 'normal' response. This belief helps us realize that, when work is challenging, there is a crisis, or when care doesn't go as expected, the response we have to that is usually our body and mind's way of making sense of it, which is what it's programmed to do. When working in demanding environments which we feel are professionally and emotionally challenging, it is more important to have this view than to label what someone is experiencing as a 'condition' in order to pathologize it.

Aside from a pandemic or a crisis occurring at work, normalizing that working in the helping profession is often emotionally intense, physically exhausting and personally challenging is, at times worthwhile. So, when we feel inadequate or have trouble forgiving ourselves for actions made (or not), we can go easy on ourselves and appreciate that others feel the same.

Common humanity isn't about normalizing poor behaviour from a colleague or accepting toxic working environments. It is recognizing that emotional suffering is part of the human experience.

Example

Mandy had just had a very difficult interaction with James, a service user she was trying to support. She came away from him and was feeling frustrated, sad and questioning whether she was making any real difference to him. She bumped into Ben, her colleague, and shared what had happened and how she was feeling.

Ben responded with: 'Yep, we've all had meetings like that, Mandy. You just need to get on with it. It's all part of being a social worker.'

Mandy couldn't just get on with it, and she didn't know how to.

Common humanity with self-compassion response:
'That sounds difficult, Mandy, and it can feel really tough when you don't feel like you're making a difference. Being a social worker means that sometimes we all feel like we aren't enough for service users. I know you do your best. If it's helpful, I can share with you some of the things I do when interactions like that leave me feeling bad.'

The first response from Ben acted to sever the connection and shared humanity. Furthermore, Mandy will potentially internalize her experience further because she cannot 'get on with it'. Hence, she may begin to feel embarrassed and ashamed and think that maybe there's something wrong with her. The-compassionate response fosters connection and common humanity and normalizes Mandy's reaction.

Mindfulness

Over the past few decades, mindfulness has grown in popularity and is used extensively as part of many therapeutic interventions. The majority of us know that it can help in numerous mental health conditions and support us when we feel overwhelmed in our day-to-day life. Jon Kabat-Zinn, founder of the mindfulness-based Stress Reduction programme, advocates for mindfulness as a process of awareness for the present moment and exploration of feelings and emotions without judgement.[8]

Although mindfulness and self-compassion are two separate practices in their own right, research demonstrates the benefits to helping professionals when they are combined. This includes reducing stress and burnout and enhancing self-compassion and empathy for patients.[9] If you're new to practising self-compassion, trying mindfulness might be a good place to start.

There are many different mindful self-compassion exercises, two of which I've outlined below if you wish to try.

Exercise: Self-compassion break

This exercise can be applied in the moment and takes only a few minutes.

Bring to mind a situation in your life that is causing you upset or some stress (not the most extreme one).

How does this situation make you feel? Where in your body do you feel the emotion? When you feel connected to the situation and associated feelings, try saying the following affirmations to yourself, either out loud or in your mind:

- 'This hurts' or 'I'm finding this stressful' – this will activate mindfulness.
- 'All of us sometimes suffer in life', 'I am not alone', 'others feel this way, too' – remember common humanity and that part of being human means we will suffer at some point; it is unavoidable.
- 'I will try to be kind to myself', 'May I be patient with myself' or 'I will forgive myself' – whatever you think is most appropriate for your situation.

Exercise: Best friend voice

Being self-compassionate involves recognizing that being imperfect and failing is inevitable, and that life will have its difficulties. However, resisting this as reality can result in feeling self-critical and often stressed. Learning to accept this with kindness and gentleness can move us closer to a more self-compassionate space.

I like this exercise below as it can help us see when our mind is being unkind to us and our inner critic is being loud. It encourages us to consider how we would treat others if they were in that situation versus how we treat ourselves. If you feel able to, it might be helpful to write down your answers to this.

- Bring to mind a time when you struggled at work. It might have been something you got wrong, a situation which didn't go as planned, or the way you behaved with a colleague or someone you were helping.
- Next, what did your mind say to you about this? Did it make judgements about you? Was it bullying you? Were the criticisms loud? What tone does this take? What are you feeling? Where in your body were you feeling it?
- Now think about a friend or a loved one coming to you. When you have that image in your mind, read out your situation, thoughts and feelings as if it were their experience.
- Imagine how you would feel when they shared this with you and your response. How would your tone be? What might you say?
- If you feel able to, write this down. Take a moment and read this through, connecting with the words and sentiment.
- Next, think about how you could use this when you're in a similar situation in the future. You might write out just a few words or a sentence to guide you at that moment to mindfully enhance your self-compassion.

Challenging our inner critic

We all have an inner critic, the voice that gives us a hard time for the decision we made or when something didn't go as expected. Its tone is rarely one of kindness, understanding and empathy. Often, it's the opposite.

We can't get rid of our inner critic. Unfortunately, it's here to stay. However, we can recognize when we are critical or negative with ourselves, the words we say, the tone we use, and how this makes us feel. Hopefully, some of the exercises so far have helped you to begin to observe your thoughts, which is the first step in learning how to have a different relationship with your inner critic.

The next step is to respond to the negative self-talk with words of understanding, using a gentle, compassionate and loving tone. You could even incorporate your 'best friend voice' from the previous exercise to help you. Words have power, and so catching how we talk to ourselves can help us heal our inner critic and begin to move to a more self-compassionate sense of self.

It might help make a plan about what to do when you notice your critical voice is loud.

Exercise: Challenging your inner critic

What has happened?
For example, *spoke rudely to a colleague.*

_____

What did you notice your inner critic said?
You're a horrible person.

_____

How did this make you feel?
Guilty, like a bad person.

_____

_____

What words of understanding and compassion could you say in response?
You were tired and in a rush. You're not a mean person. Go to your colleague and apologize for what you said.

_____

_____

11

Navigating toxic workplaces

Over my years of providing psychological support to staff and coaching leaders in healthcare, I have witnessed the ripple effect of toxic behaviours in a workplace on the organization, teams and individuals, as well as on those they serve. What might have started as something small, like gossiping about a colleague, soon caught traction, severing connections among colleagues and causing fragmented services. The final result may be a hostile environment that significantly compromises the staff's mental wellbeing and the quality of care that patients receive.

Some research[1] suggests that toxic workplaces can fall into four areas:

Toxic behaviours of co-workers	Toxic behaviours of managers	Toxic social-structural factors	Toxic climate
Gossiping Aggression Humiliation Negative acts Incivility	Narcissism & egoism Anger outburst & aggression Abusive Negative jokes & humiliation Favouritism Politics & favouring	Unreasonable overwork hours or tasks Career obstacles Unfair evaluations & politics Ergonomics & physical conditions	Low trust Work stressors Discrimination

Learning how to manage this when working with challenging colleagues, rather than getting caught up in or contributing to this, can protect our wellbeing. Francoise Mathieu, Executive Director of TEND and the author of *The Compassion Fatigue Workbook*, describes toxic workplaces as an organizational form of compassion fatigue caused by vicarious trauma and compassion fatigue experienced by some of our most exhausted colleagues.

Christine Porath is an associate professor at the McDonough School of Business at Georgetown University and is the author of *Mastering Civility*. For over 20 years, along with colleagues, she has surveyed the impact of rudeness on thousands of staff across numerous industries, including health and social care. Most recipients of rudeness lose time worrying about the rude interactions they have encountered with colleagues. The quality of their work suffers, and almost half of people surveyed reduce their time at work, with many affected staff taking their frustrations out on service users. Incivility affects more than just the recipient; it affects everyone and dilutes the care being provided.

Some suggestions below are outlined to help you begin to think about ways to protect yourself from the negative effects of toxic workplaces.

Connecting with others

The primary support for staff within organizations often comes from colleagues and managers. Social support from them can reduce stress and perceived work overload;[2] therefore, finding those in our workplace who are supportive can positively impact our wellbeing. The psychiatrist Bessel van der Kolk, author of *The Body Keeps the Score*, shared about the importance of feeling safe with others and the fundamental importance of this to an individual's mental health.

- **Try to be inclusive to new members of staff**, particularly students or junior members of the team. When someone new starts, do you introduce yourself? Tell them where the canteen is? Show them where the toilet is? Try to be welcoming?
- **Being kind.** It sounds simple, doesn't it? Yet when we feel overwhelmed, stressed and tired, being kind might be something that goes out the window. We don't have to *feel* kind to *do* acts of kindness, but they require us to make a conscious effort and intend to do them. They don't necessarily need to be labour- and time-intensive. They could be simple acts of kindness.

- **Manners:** say good morning/afternoon/evening to colleagues. Say 'thank you' and 'please'. Acknowledge and thank a team when its members have worked hard, worked well together or have overcome a difficult obstacle.

- **Eye contact:** when a colleague looks stressed, catch their eye, and making a small gesture; it could be a slight nod of your head or smile. What you're saying is: I see you; I'm acknowledging your stress; and I'm with you. If you're able to, later on, you could share with them that they looked stressed and enquire how they are.

Learning to say 'no'

Inadequate staffing levels in health and social care can rarely meet many organizations' demands, leaving staff overworked and their mental wellbeing compromised.[3, 4] Setting boundaries protects our wellbeing. Yet, when we see colleagues overstretched, what I see many people doing is more, not less, and the system around us allows this, even expects this.

However, turning someone down when they request our help is a skill, so telling someone to be assertive won't make them feel more assertive. Here are some ways that might help you to say 'no':

- **Just give one reason.** Try not to blame something or someone else. If you feel able to give an honest response, then do so, rather than providing a litany of reasons or excuses, as you're under so much pressure; you're behind with your work; you don't have the time. Try giving just one reason: 'I would like to be able to help, but I'm not able to this time because…'
- **Stand firm.** Many of us might feel railroaded into agreeing to do something we don't want to. Do you get anxious or worried when you've said what you want to happen, but someone continues to push their agenda? If so, use some of the strategies we've already discussed, maybe breathe mindfully, or carry out some positive self-talk: 'You can do this.' Then deliver, 'I hear what you're saying, and you need some help with sorting this, but I'm just not able to do it.' Try to stay calm and repeat what you've said if the railroading continues.

- **Alternatives to 'no'.** If you don't feel able to say 'no' outright, you could say, 'Can you leave that with me?' 'I'll check my schedule and get back to you; 'let me think if I can help with that and I'll let you know.' When asked to do overtime or take on another project, whatever it might be, some of us might feel caught 'off-guard' and so in the moment say 'yes' without realizing what it is we are committing to. These phrases act to buy some time, so you can go and think of the response you might like to make.

Exercise: Learning to say 'no'

When do you notice you find it difficult to be assertive at work?

_____

_____

What does your mind say and your body feel during these interactions?

_____

_____

If you struggle to say 'no', what else could you say or do?

_____

_____

When might you try this out?

_____

_____

What might get in the way of you doing this?

_____

_____

_____

_____

Beware of negative people

Small talk and gossip are two different things. Small talk is a way of socially connecting with others through a polite conversation about unimportant topics, while gossip typically involves sharing information about others, often without their knowledge. One breeds connection, and the other breeds toxicity.

Although you can't always avoid being around colleagues who gossip, are critical, bitter, complain or engage in negativity, try to reduce the time you have with them. It can feel draining to be in the company of people who behave in these ways.

Finding your voice

Brené Brown, a research professor at the University of Houston, has studied emotions, particularly vulnerability and courage. I think of her work when witnessing or coaching individuals to step up and take a risk to speak out about something important to them. For many of us, this can take immense courage, particularly if our working environment isn't psychologically safe and we can't know the outcome. This is vulnerability, and many of us have stories that our head tells us what it means to be vulnerable: 'It's a sign of weakness', 'It's giving someone else the upper hand over you', 'People won't respect you.'

I have witnessed countless acts of courage in my work, none of which was done without the person connecting with their vulnerability. It can feel hard doing this because it is a risk that we take: to step up and speak out when we don't know what the outcome will be.

Getting started with knowing how to approach a conversation that you suspect feels difficult might feel hard. The following suggestions might help to support you as you think about how to frame a difficult discussion:

- **What do you want to say?** Be clear and concise about exactly what you want to say.
- **What do you want the outcome to be?** This does not necessarily mean that it will happen. However, being clear on this

will help you and the person you're speaking with know what you are asking for.

- **How do you want to say it?** If you don't feel comfortable, or this is a new skill you're learning, practise the conversation with someone you feel safe being around. Play out the tone you want to use that is respectful and kind. Connect with the part of you that feels strong and confident.

It might help to write some of this down or practise it with someone you trust.

Nurturing our young

Entering the health and social care systems as a student can be incredibly overwhelming. Gruelling exams to test technical abilities and breadth of knowledge, although beneficial, don't necessarily provide students with the necessary skills to navigate complex and challenging working environments.

Staff shortages have long been a workforce issue in health and social care. With an increase in the world population, the World Health Organization (WHO) has projected a global shortage of 2.3 million doctors by 2030.[5] To address the shortages across health and social care professions, many nursing, midwifery, medical and social work schools are making extra places for more students on their programmes. Although this is a welcome step, a potential shortfall will remain within some professions because retaining graduates when they are qualified is another problem to face.

'We Eat Our Young' is a common idiom used within some healthcare professions to describe the bullying behaviours experienced primarily by junior staff and students from their senior colleagues. Many beginning their careers experience horizontal violence (overt and covert non-physical hostility), such as bickering, scapegoating, sabotaging, undermining and criticism.[6] All this can have a profound psychological impact on them, so much so that they consider leaving their profession.

Experiences of rudeness, abusive language and humiliation from colleagues were the most commonly experienced forms of horizontal violence experienced by nurses in their first year of practice. The psychological fallout of this was that they felt undervalued and emotionally neglected. Only a small portion of those who experienced a distressing incident received formal counselling, and less than half of the incidents were reported.[7]

As previously discussed, UK midwives' emotional wellbeing is worse than that of midwives in other countries, with many experiencing high levels of burnout, stress, anxiety, and depression.[8] Currently, the attrition rates are greatest in the NHS during the first two years post qualifying.[9] How staff imagined their role as a qualified midwife might have been, and the reality of what it is, may not match. It might be due to a lack of support, overstretched resources, and an inability to provide the care they've been trained to do.

Resilience training has been hailed as one possible solution to prepare students (and the existing workforce) to cope better to work in emotionally intense environments. I don't have a problem with resilience training per se; rather, it's the message that it conveys to staff, particularly when it is offered as the only option to support their wellbeing.

In the UK, some NHS job specifications specify medical graduates to have proved they are resilient, that is, they can recover quickly from difficult situations. It is now taught as part of the curriculum in medical schools. The resilience narrative implies a need for us to be tougher and more malleable, accepting and compliant of a deeply flawed healthcare system. This doesn't consider what needs to change to make the system resilient to support those it employs better. It also makes a dangerous assumption that we all experience our working environment in similar ways. This is not the case. We are all too familiar with the inequalities that play out due to gender, race and culture within the helping profession. My belief is that, when the environmental conditions of psychological safety and nurture are in place, we are better able to develop our resilience to protect ourselves in the challenges we face at work.

By 2022, there will be approximately 65,000 social workers trained in healthcare, substance misuse, or mental health in the United States,[10] with a significant focus on developing integrated health delivery and interprofessional team practice. Although students were more motivated to develop their clinical skills within many of the training programmes, by one year postgraduation, they identified that leadership preparation for system-level change was important.[11] Every student has the potential to become a leader. Our responsibility, both on training programmes and in practice, is to foster the right conditions to be the best practitioners possible.

There is an obvious irony here that we don't tend to 'care' for those working in caring professions. In few other areas of the helping profession are staff so ill-equipped to manage the emotional and physical challenges of their area of work. We bring our whole selves to work. Given that the workplace is often where we disburse most of our energy, being encouraged to keep emotions away from this space sets us up to fail because this is impossible to do.

There is a human response that being involved in a distressing event evokes and that will impact each of us differently. Normalizing this and creating safe spaces within teams and organizations that support and 'hold' us when this happens is essential. This requires a two-prong approach, giving students and existing staff the tools to help themselves when working in a challenging, under-resourced, and overstretched system and addressing why these exist in the first place. Teaching us about negotiating relationships, employment rights, addressing bullying or intimidating behaviours, and raising concerns without fear of reprisal or retribution would forearm us all. When we fail to train students to navigate a complex environment and protect themselves in their role, we not only are damaging them, but we are losing our future leaders.

Exercise: Coping with feelings

Use the following questions as a guide to support you as you think about how you feel when feelings arise at work that you find difficult to manage, how you might respond to these, and what you might do differently.

What situations, people, or events trigger emotions you find difficult to cope with at work?

_____

_____

_____

_____

_____

What does your mind say and your body feel?

_____

_____

_____

_____

_____

How could you respond in a way that is kind to yourself?

_____

_____

_____

_____

_____

12

Unlocking the power of positivity

At some point, life is hard for us all, and some certainly have it harder than others. Have you ever wondered about the different responses people have to life's difficulties? Some feel crushed by hardship, others cope relatively well, and then some seem to come back even stronger than before. There are copious research studies that have demonstrated that positivity is the ingredient that helps people bounce back from adversity. It doesn't mean that they walk around every day with a smile on their face and are entirely impervious to distress; instead, it's how they respond that's the key. When we feel swallowed up by life and difficult emotions, positivity can be our lifeline. The practice of positivity is not the same as the rhetoric to 'just think positive'. This is learning the skill of positivity and implementing it into our lives.

Barbara Fredrickson is a Professor of Psychology, and her ground-breaking research into positivity has been revolutionary in helping people change their relationship with negative emotions. She has discovered that when our blood pressure rises due to feelings like anxiety, we have a 'reset' button for these spikes: our own positive emotions. Alongside restoring normal blood pressure levels, good feelings quieten our heart and flush out our difficult feelings.[1, 2]

Those who bounce back from minor everyday stressors in significant life events display more emotional complexity when facing stressors. It's more complex because, when they are faced with adversity, their feelings of negativity sit alongside positivity, so they feel the impact of what has happened. Still, they don't get enveloped by it. Working in the helping professions means that we might have multiple stressors, perhaps daily, which affect our mental wellbeing. Still, positivity might have the power to pull us out of a negative abyss. We all have colleagues who, when stress is high at work, can generate positivity themselves. Take the following example:

June is a social worker in a small team and has recently been diagnosed with cancer. She has a large caseload, and so when she goes off on sick leave and her work is distributed between her two colleagues, both have different responses.

Rachel's response: 'I've even more work now. I was already overstretched. It's going to be so stressful. I'm not sure how I will cope.'

Michelle's response: 'This will be tough, but there are some conditions here I've never worked with before. I'm going to learn loads over the next few months.

You can hear the emotional weight the extra work might have on Rachel, whereas, although Michelle also acknowledges that the next few months will be difficult, she can also see opportunities where she might benefit.

When we experience negativity, it can be pervasive, infiltrating our thoughts and relationships and connections with others. They can fertilize other emotions such as bitterness and anger, which can compromise our health. In different parts of our brain, the positive and negative systems are organized differently and potentially develop differently throughout our lifetimes. That means that, when we are in a spiral of thinking critically about ourselves or being pessimistic, this reinforces and strengthens the neural circuits that support these functions. If our focus is on being kind, on self-compassion, gratitude and compassion for others, these circuits will strengthen.

According to Fredrickson's Positivity Ratio, it doesn't take very much to tip us from being negative into a more positive state. In her best-selling book *Positivity*, which was the culmination of 20 years of research, she stated that people who have positive emotions in a ratio of 3:1, in relation to negative emotions, are more likely to flourish. Although others have disputed the ratio figure, the overall view remains – that if positive rather than negative influences surround us, people are likely to enjoy their life, help others, and cope better when under stress.

Working in the helping professions can significantly compromise our mental wellbeing due to hostile working cultures. The team and organization do not necessarily create these. Rather, there could be many negative interactions daily. For example, being verbally abused by those we are trying to support; being physically assaulted by patients in our workplaces; being spat at; a colleague being rude to us. Such interactions provoke adverse reactions in us, such as anger or anxiety.

Over the decades, positive psychology has expanded. Interventions have been developed to encourage people to identify and develop their own positive emotions and experiences. Although there is a range of interventions available, two evidence-based positive psychology interventions that don't require an extensive skillset but do demand an intention and commitment are: practising gratitude[3] and encouraging random acts of kindness.[4]

Practising gratitude

Gratitude is so much more than feeling thankful. It's a deeper appreciation for someone or something that creates longer-lasting positivity. Gratitude is a social emotion in that it can strengthen existing relationships or foster new ones, serving a biological purpose. Over the past three decades, the research into the benefits of practising gratitude has gained significant traction, and the results are compelling.

Simple gratitude practices like saying 'thank you' or a kind gesture has a long-lasting effect on our brain and nervous system.[5] There are two key neurotransmitters (serotonin and dopamine) that are responsible for our emotions and that make us feel good when expressing and receiving gratitude. When released, they enhance our mood almost immediately and make us feel happier. Also, evidence has indicated that the part of our brain responsible for emotional experiences (the limbic system) gets activated with feelings of gratitude, particularly the two main areas (the hippocampus and the amygdala) that regulate emotions, memory and bodily functioning.[6] By stimulating our brain's reward centre through gratitude practices, we alter our view of ourselves and the world. So, by setting an intention to practise gratitude every day, we can strengthen these neural pathways, creating a more positive and grateful part of ourselves.

I previously mentioned our brains being hard-wired for predictability and making associations quickly. The same is true when we get into a spiral of negative thinking. The more negative thoughts go round in our minds, the more our brains will be fine-tuned to subconsciously focus on negativity. While many emotions can be experienced alongside one another such as grief and happiness or guilt and hope, it's tough to hold negative and positive information simultaneously. Therefore, we can train our brains to selectively attend to positive thoughts and emotions, alleviating our feelings of anxiety and worry.

Working in the helping profession is stressful. We know that. Many studies have reported that the practice of gratitude reduces our levels of the stress hormone (cortisol).[7] While reducing stress hormones and managing the autonomic nervous system functions, gratitude has also been shown to reduce symptoms of anxiety and depression. When we experience gratitude, this positively affects the brain's activity (prefrontal cortex) responsible for managing emotions like guilt and shame. So, for people working in highly stressful environments that are more vulnerable to vicarious trauma and moral injury, this can be significantly beneficial. We are better supported to deal with these emotional setbacks and negative incidents.

Exercise: Practising gratitude

If you have only 10–90 seconds:

- Be generous with your thank-yous and pleases to colleagues and patients/clients/services users. This requires you to actively watch for things others do that are helpful, thoughtful and kind.
- Take a moment; breathe in fully; exhale fully; and appreciate something at that moment, for example 'I'm grateful for this coffee' or 'I'm grateful I'm able to take a lunch break.'
- At the end of the working day, share one thing with your team you are grateful for, for example 'I'm grateful that, although the Emergency Department was busy, that we worked together to reduce the waiting times for patients.'

If you have 30 minutes:

- Gratitude partner: find someone you can practise your daily gratitude with; it could be a colleague, friend, spouse or child.

Ask questions and share the things that you're grateful for to cultivate and strengthen feelings of gratitude.

- Create a gratitude jar: have a stack of small blank notes beside an empty jar, and each day, ask staff to write down one thing they are feeling grateful for. It could be that, once a week, someone takes a collection of them and reads them out to their team. You could create one for your family, too.
- After a hard day at work, it might feel like there wasn't a lot to be grateful for. Asking yourself the following questions might help you to generate gratitude:
  - What was the best thing that happened today?
  - What made me smile?
  - What moved or touched me today?

If you have 55–60 minutes:

- Write thank you notes or letters. We all have people in our lives who have played a big part in helping us through difficult times; they are always there for us when we need it; they always step in when we need childcare, or whatever it might be that we need. Write them a note or letter expressing your gratitude to them.
- Start a gratitude journal. Studies have shown that writing down all of the people, experiences and things in our life that we're grateful for can positively impact on our mental wellbeing. Below are some suggestions on how to prepare and maintain a gratitude journal:[8]
  - Commit to daily practice.
  - Set aside some time (e.g. early in the morning or right before bedtime) and journal your gratitude at the same time every day.
  - Go through the previous pages and recollect the good things that happened to you in the past.
  - When filling the journal, try to be as detailed as you can. Record every little thing associated with the person or the incident you are offering your gratitude to.
  - Make your journal attractive. Use colourful pens, stickers or craft papers to give the gratitude journal an exciting look. Make journaling more of an experience than a daily practice.

Random acts of kindness

When we let a car that is waiting to get out of a junction go first, we hold the door open for someone coming behind us, or we make a colleague a longed-for hot drink, our actions are met with gratitude from the receiver, and we usually feel pretty good about ourselves. These small acts of kindness create a warm feeling inside us because of the 'love hormone' oxytocin.

It is well established that oxytocin plays a part in forming trust and forming social bonds, as well as when we have sex, and when mothers touch, smell and connect with their babies. When oxytocin is released, it benefits us physically, as it lowers our blood pressure, our heart rate and improves our quality of sleep. The giving and receiving of simple acts of kindness triggers a part of our brain that regulates all bodily mechanisms, of which sleep is one. Simple acts of kindness activated by hypothalamic regulation are more likely to support us to have a deeper and healthier sleep.[9]

Psychologically, engaging in random acts of kindness that trigger oxytocin tends to make us more trusting, generous and friendlier towards others. Studies have also indicated that these acts release the feel-good neurotransmitter dopamine, giving us a euphoric feeling, and have been linked with causing what's termed as a 'helper's high'. Besides oxytocin and dopamine being boosted when we engage in deeds of kindness, another neurotransmitter called serotonin is released, regulating our mood.

Like most things, doing single acts of kindness isn't enough to sustain our physical and mental wellbeing. We need to incorporate it into our daily practice to gain the most benefits. I've listed a few simple acts of kindness below to inspire you. It would be great if you took these and added to them, created your own, and shared the inspiration with others.

- Pay someone a compliment.
- Send someone a book you think they might enjoy.
- Tell colleagues how much your team values them.
- Buy a colleague a coffee.
- Make cakes for your team.

- Ask a colleague how they are feeling and make the time to listen.

Exercise: Random acts of kindness

List the random acts of kindness you could action:

_____

_____

_____

_____

_____

Over the next four weeks, list some of the acts of kindness you can show to:
Yourself:

_____

_____

_____

Colleagues:

_____

_____

_____

Loved ones:

_____

_____

_____

13

The magic is inside you

In the introductory chapter, I shared the power that the vagus nerve has. It is a significant part of the parasympathetic (rest–digest state) branch of the autonomic nervous system and is a 'family of neural pathways'. Having a higher vagal tone can support us globally, particularly in challenging work environments, like health and social care, because these daily experiences can overwhelm our ventral vagal system. So, by having a higher vagal tone, we can better connect with ourselves and others and return to a calmer state more quickly when exposed to stress.

What if you could learn to use your neurobiology so you can draw upon it when you need it the most? Our autonomic nervous system responds to two competing needs, which can shift in moments: to survive and to be social. Survival is the only objective when in a state of protection, which makes change and connection difficult. In contrast, health and renewal are possible in a state of connection. So, balancing the need to survive with the want to connect is tricky.

Professor Stephen Porges developed the polyvagal theory (PVT), which provides us with a neurobiological framework to help us understand what is happening in our body and our nervous system, particularly how our sense of safety, danger or threat can impact our behaviours. Throughout this book, we have discussed how connecting with your body and how it is feeling, and interpreting what it is telling you, is necessary to support you when you need it the most. Deb Dana is a clinician and consultant who adapted PVT in her work with complex trauma. She reiterates that, in order to reshape our autonomic nervous system in a new way, we need to be able first to identify our autonomic states: collapse or shutdown (dorsal vagal), fight or flight (sympathetic), and safe and connected (ventral vagal). Connecting with our different states might feel difficult, so to give you an idea of how someone might experience these, I've provided some examples below:

Collapse or shutdown (dorsal vagal)

Becky returned home after a hectic and long day at work. She was juggling many different projects, rushed back to spend some time with her family, and made a nutritious meal. While it was cooking in the oven, and the kids were preoccupied, she thought she would catch up with some emails that had built up over the day. Becky realized 30 minutes had passed, rushed into the kitchen, opened the oven, and the dinner had dried out; it was ruined. Becky felt like this was a complete disaster. 'I'm finished' was what she said, not really knowing what that meant, and she sat on her own, feeling numb. After 20 minutes or so, she got up, sorted out the food that was baked on to the dish, and prepared an alternative. The overwhelming demands of the day were already too much, so the dried-out dinner was the final straw for her autonomic system.

Fight or flight (sympathetic)

Kevin, Amir's junior, had a query about a patient he wasn't sure about, so he went to speak to his senior colleague. As Kevin approached Amir writing his notes, Amir looked up at him and returned to his notes, saying nothing. Kevin went on to share what he needed, and his colleague continued to ignore him. Kevin could feel his blood beginning to boil at the dismissal. At that moment, he unleashed his anger verbally onto his colleague and stormed off, furious. When Kevin was at school, he had been bullied and had learned growing up not to be noticed. However, as an adult, when he feels someone is ignoring or dismissing his experience, he is primed and ready to fight. Although his colleague had been rude, Kevin could see when he had calmed down that it was his previous experience that had been triggered during the exchange with his colleague.

Safe and connected (ventral vagal)

Simone had been involved in treating a patient at work whose care hadn't gone as expected, and sadly he died. Her place of work suggested she take some time off. A week or so later, Simone was still feeling low in mood and sad. As she was sitting outside, she wondered whether she would ever be the same again. Simone closed her eyes and imagined her mum being there with her, holding her, stroking her hair, providing reassurance. She could imagine her mum there with her, the smell of her, the gentle tone of her voice, and soft but familiar touch. Although she still felt sad and low, she also had a sense of peace and hope that came over her and a feeling of hope that she would be okay.

Exercise: Connecting with your autonomic states

Recall memories that might help you connect with the three states and write a few sentences or words to help you recognize signs when you shift into each of them.

- **Collapse or shutdown** (dorsal states can sometimes feel numb, floppy or foggy)

  _____

  _____

- **Fight or flight** (sympathetic states might feel energixing and charged)

  _____

  _____

- **Safe and connected** (ventral vagal states might feel calm, passionate, joyful)

  _____

  _____

Just as our needs change throughout the day, so do the inter-actions between our three autonomic states. Given that many behaviours generated by the autonomic nervous system are not conscious, many of our actions are automatic and adaptive. So, when you're trying to get in touch with these states, it might be helpful to think about situations or circumstances when you found yourself questioning why you behaved as you did or if someone said you 'overreacted' in some way. Think about how many times during the day your feelings change. If there is a change in your feeling, that's a good indicator there has been an autonomic change.

Understandably, when I speak with staff groups about finding ways to look after themselves when working in challenging environments, one of the most common barriers is being time-poor. So, like most of the exercises in this book, trying to incorporate these techniques into your daily routine and practising them when away from work will support you more when you need to call on them when you're in your role.

Music

Sound, music and singing impact the way we feel. Music can be a way to connect us to safety. It can evoke lots of different emotions in us, from happiness to sadness and even distress. Listening to or creating music is classed as an autonomic exercise because it involves our head and facial muscles, and our middle ear muscles which support listening.[1]

The vagus nerve is connected to the vocal cords and muscles at the back of our throat. The vibrations from singing, humming, chanting and gargling stimulate our vagus nerve, and all have been shown to increase our heart rate variability and vagal tone.[2]

You could try:

- listening to music on your way to/from work;
- humming/singing while you're walking along the corridor or while you're at your computer;
- gargling water before swallowing it.

Deep breathing

Most people take about 10 to 14 breaths each minute. When we are in a fight/flight state, our breathing shifts to our chest, but we can become anxious when our breathing stays there.

Learning to breath more slowly, taking about six breaths over one minute, and deeply from your belly, where your diaphragm is, can stimulate the vagus nerve, supporting a state of relaxation.

Try the following:

1 Sit down, in a comfortable position, with your eyes closed or opened with a softened gaze.
2 Begin by taking several long slow breaths, breathing in fully and exhaling fully, long and slow. Notice the gentle rise of your belly on the in-breath and the relaxing letting go of the out-breath.
3 Allow your breath to find its natural rhythm. Don't try to force it in any way.

Laughing

Any type of laughter has been shown to stimulate diaphragmatic breathing, which, as described above, triggers activation of our vagus nerve. It is believed that our body is unable to differentiate between assimilated laughter and laughing at something we find genuinely funny.[3] So, whether we recall a funny memory, watch something comical, or start to laugh, these are all ways to tone our vagus nerve.

Exercise: Using anchors

When you're activated and are heading towards fight/flight or shutdown mode, anchors are a great way to draw you back to your ventral vagal state and help you stay there. With regular practice, anchors can strengthen your ability to manage difficult emotions, using who, what, where and when categories. Try to write as many examples as you can.

- **Who?** Make a list of the people (and the pets) in your life who make you feel safe and content when you're with them. This list could also include those who are no longer alive or are spiritual beings.

_____

_____

_____

- **What?** Think about things you do that make you feel alive, nourished or joyful. It could be something simple like watering your plants or going for a walk. Again, think of the micro-moments that you feel grateful for.

_____

_____

_____

- **Where?** These are the places where you feel connected and safe. It could be somewhere in your home, community, neighbourhood, or a place you can access at work.

_____

_____

_____

- **When?** Recollect the memories when you felt safe. It could be moments or more extended periods.

_____

_____

_____

14
Summary

Applying self-care strategies on their own is not enough to protect your mental wellbeing at work and safeguard you from the impact of trauma, burnout, compassion fatigue and moral injury. First, you need to connect with yourself and know what signs in your body and mind indicate that you need to stop, put the brakes on, and tend to yourself. The right connections need to be in place to create and maintain habits to support your mental wellbeing successfully. For an action to become an automatic habit, some suggest that it takes 66 days of practice. While missing one day here and there won't detrimentally affect the success of you developing the habit and integrating self-care practices into your life, continued support is essential. Rather than focusing on the outcome of the goal, imagine the person you want to be, for example, you could imagine yourself calmer, mentally healthier or happier. Think about all the effort you will undoubtedly contribute to supporting those in your role, and consider how much do you input to yourself, not only in the service to help others but because you deserve to be cared for too.

In Part II of this book, I will discuss how your behaviours can indicate what you might need, the barriers to reaching out for help when you need it, and treatment options to support you in optimizing your mental wellbeing.

Part II
RECEIVING SUPPORT

Stress is a normal response to difficult situations and working in challenging environments. It can even be helpful to us in the moment. The purpose of this section is not to provide a checklist of signs and symptoms you might be experiencing (though these are covered in the introductory Chapter 15). Instead, Part II aims to help you think about when your usual amount of stress tips into feelings that render you physically or psychologically unwell, and you experience burnout, compassion fatigue, moral injury or psychological trauma.

15

Behaviours as symptoms

We feel feelings in our bodies, not in our heads. So, tuning into our body can be hugely advantageous in supporting us to know when our emotions are becoming more severe. However, for many people, connecting with how they feel is foreign, or they are disconnected from their body in some way. This could be for many different reasons: it doesn't feel safe to be connected with your body; it feels frightening or painful; or you've never been taught how to listen to what your body is saying. Whatever the reason, other indicators, like our behaviours, let us know that we might need support, but we need to be open to seeing them. Three of these behaviours include defensive practice, depersonalized care and substance misuse.

Defensive practice

The infestation of fear among health and social care professions is rising, and within both industries fear impacts differently on practices. Feeling fearful is not necessarily something that is always experienced on a conscious level, so you might not even be aware you are frightened. It is something that could be lurking in the back of our minds. Fear can breed rampantly within teams and develop in us slowly over time. It can develop by us observing the impact of repercussions on colleagues, hearing others' stories, and reading about them, for example, in the media or professional regulator newsletters. The fear might not even be ours; it could be passed down to us by colleagues, mentors, supervisors or our organizations. By observing our behaviours at work, we can gain insights into how we might be feeling and into those indicators we might need to seek support.

Within healthcare

Fear of consequences has been cited as a pivotal concern for healthcare professionals, particularly physicians and nurses. There is significant variability between these groups in error-reporting behaviours and the fear of repercussions they face.[1] However, the rise of anxiety and defensive practice of medicine has been linked to lack of resources, and increasing demands from patients, and has been directly linked to an increase in fear of liability claims and lawsuits.[2]

Behaviours that are indicative of defensive medicine fall into two categories: negative and positive defensive medicine. Negative defensive medicine attempts to avoid high-risk patients or procedures, whereas assurance behaviours, or positive defensive medicine, involve ordering extra diagnostic tests, procedures, overprescribing medication, or unnecessary hospital visits.

Both avoidance and assurance behaviours attempt to minimize exposure to malpractice liability. However, within medicolegal cases, there are presently more lawsuits based on alleged acts of omission on the medical professional's part than other types of errors. This possibly serves to incentivise practitioners to implement more assurance behaviours to mitigate potential legal risk.[3,4] Below is an example of a more subtle but relatively common positive defensive medicine action.

Dr Fong is a GP. Each appointment of his morning had overrun, and he knew that leaving on time was not possible. He had worked through his lunch break in an attempt to get through the jobs on his list. Dr Fong's next appointment was with a mother who came in with her eight-year-old child. She described her child's symptoms, and she was pretty distressed, wanting to know what was wrong with her child; she was sleep-deprived, having been up during the past few nights with him. Dr Fong examined the child, and it was evident he had a cold and possible ear infection, so he advised the mother to ensure her child had plenty of fluids, rest and pain relief. However, she was adamant he needed antibiotics. He didn't think this was necessary, but she persisted, was becoming tearful, and was very forceful. Dr Fong was aware she had previously put a complaint about his colleague into the practice manager. He prescribed antibiotics.

Defensive medicine harms patients by putting them through unnecessary procedures and hospitalization, which might distress them and their families. Apart from the obvious increase in costs that defensive medicine creates,[5] these practices also negatively affect the nurse/doctor–patient relationship. Not only does it generate mistrust in patients, but physicians regard patients as complainants.[6]

As discussed, practising defensively is linked to fear; however, there are many reasons why fear is present, and needs addressing. Fear could result from pressure and could be a combination of both direct and indirect factors that contribute to creating fear and defensive practice in staff, such as:

- having been involved in litigation or complaint proceedings previously;
- witnessing or hearing the experiences of colleagues;
- being involved in care that has not gone as expected;
- patients you perceive as 'demanding';
- organizational or system processes.

Alongside litigation, physicians fear blame, liability, estrangement from peers, and poor publicity. Therefore, reporting of medical errors is significantly hampered due to these.[7,8] Evidence suggests that nurses tend to be more forthcoming about reporting medical errors, but fear disciplinary action from their supervisors, managers or physicians.[9,10] Additionally, they worry that, if the errors are noted in their files, this will restrict their career progression.[11] These behaviours shine a spotlight on the organization and the system that healthcare staff work in. To remedy this issue requires a significant culture shift, where staff learn to practise safely and share when care does not go as expected, without fear of retribution from the organization or the patients.

The idea of shared decision-making is not a new concept in healthcare. It has been defined as 'an approach where clinicians and patients share the best available evidence when faced with the task of making decisions, and where patients are supported to consider options, to achieve informed preferences'.[12] It is based on the premise that patients are the experts on what matters most to them and healthcare professionals hold medical expertise.[13]

In 2016, the 'Choosing Wisely' campaign was launched in the UK and was part of a global initiative to improve the conversations between patients and their doctors and nurses. It listed 40 tests and treatments that are unlikely to benefit patients as well as principles to encourage patients to get the best from conversations with their doctors and nurses by asking four questions:

1 What are the benefits?
2 What are the risks?
3 What are the alternatives?
4 What if I do nothing?

Practising defensively takes you away from shared decision-making and possibly the professional code many of you have, which is to provide the best care possible and do no harm. That said, if you are practising defensively, it will be a symptom of something else, and it is important to be curious and learn what drives that behaviour and to look for the support you might need to practise differently.

Due to significant pressure for practitioners to see more patients in a shorter time, with fewer resources and many staff having to spend increasing amounts of time inputting patient data digitally, the relationship between the patient and the practitioner becomes significantly diluted. It has been suggested[14] that some ways to support medical staff from practising defensively include:

• reaffirming the importance of clinical reasoning;
• increasing time spent with patients directly;
• organizational support for staff who have experienced adverse patient events.

The onus to support staff to stop engaging in defensive actions does not rest exclusively with you. On the contrary, what is required is a shift in the organization to create a culture of learning, rather than blame, and where practitioners feel able to share when they have been involved in care that has not gone as expected. We need cultures that nurture staff and where psychological safety is embedded in teams, policies and organizational procedures.

Within social care

Defensive practice within social work practice has been defined as 'practices which are deliberately chosen to protect the professional worker, at the possible expense of the wellbeing of the client'.[15] Similar to defensive medicine practices, some behaviours include unnecessary intervention or the avoidance engagement or action, for example:

- removing a child needlessly;
- not attending supervision meetings or rescheduling them;
- excessively documenting practice;
- restraining from intervention, for example not returning a child home when it is appropriate to do so;
- avoiding challenging service users.

These behaviours protect the worker from being held responsible and blamed, and they might be seen as obvious signs of defensive practice. However, being aware of subtle actions of defensiveness is essential. Intervening when you notice these will help to prevent you from becoming desensitized to this way of practice. Here is an example of subtle defensive action:

> Graeme was driving to meet Bill, a service user living on his own. Graeme could feel the heaviness and dread of seeing Bill, who was always so grumpy, argumentative and cantankerous. Graeme was tired, and he just didn't feel up to trying to engage Bill today. As he approached Bill's house, he knocked on the door ever so softly. He waited a few minutes, and there was no response. He tried again, and still there was no response. Graeme got back into his car, relieved he wasn't seeing Bill. He knew Bill would never have heard him knocking that gently, but he just couldn't face it.

Over the years, the social work profession has drawn considerable negativity from the UK media, particularly when serious case reviews have been publicized. For example, in 2009, in the UK, a 17-month baby named Peter Connolly found dead in his cot, and during his short life he had suffered more than 50 injuries. Investigations reported that over eight months, social workers, doctors and police had seen him 60 times, but their actions had been inadequate to protect him. The media furore that ensued launched a petition to dismiss all social workers involved and was signed by 1.4 million people.[16] Although defensive practice is present to varying degrees across all social work areas, it appears more pronounced here due to the high-profile nature of child protection. This case and many other high-profile tragedies involving children have contributed to social workers engaging in defensive practices as a means of self-protection.

Apart from negative media attention, systemic and organizational factors have been identified as contributing to defensive practice in social work, including:[17,18,19,20]

- stringent reviews, inspections audits and managerial inspection;
- need to manage perceived risk to individual staff and the organization of service users;
- managing perceived risk to service users;
- need to adhere to rules, legislation and policies.

Social care staff protect themselves for many reasons. Uncovering these reasons and openly having dialogues about them is a start to ensuring they come to work and feel fulfilled in their roles. However, similarly to healthcare staff, working in cultures that foster learning rather than repercussions will help social workers feel that they can speak out without fear of retribution.

When guidelines are used as rules, it serves to hamper our creativity in developing proper person-centred care. Furthermore, it reduces our confidence and belief that we can manage risk with service users and make the necessary decisions. Guidelines are just this: a guide that supports us to make judgements in our roles. Relying solely on them won't result in us having relationships with service users with minimal risk. Whether it's health or social care we work in, we serve people in our roles. This requires us to connect with them as individuals, and the system in which we work also requires them to connect with us as individuals. The common thread that runs throughout this is a connection with ourselves and those we support.

Exercise: Are you practising defensively?

What are subtle and obvious signs that you might be practising defensively?

Subtle signs: _____

_____

Obvious signs: _____

_____

Recall a time when your actions were defensive. What were you feeling at that time?

_____

_____

Rather than the action you took, what could you have done to manage the emotions you were experiencing?

_____

_____

What other actions could you have taken, rather than defensive?

_____

_____

What do you need in place to practise less defensively?

_____

_____

If this is not possible currently, are there alternative ways to support yourself?

_____

_____

Depersonalized care

Working in health and social care requires us to be in professional relationships with those we support and care for, sometimes at the most challenging times in their lives. Part of our role involves being able to recognize the emotions of those we support and to respond appropriately. As discussed in the introductory chapter, there is a significant overlap of burnout with other experiences such as compassion fatigue, depression, anxiety and psychological trauma in staff. Alongside exhaustion and reduced personal accomplishment in work, depersonalization of care is a clear sign of burnout in staff. Depersonalization is the core interpersonal dimension of burnout and has the most significant impact on patient care outcomes and increased complaints.[21]

High levels of emotional exhaustion increase depersonalization of patients, service users and clients. Some groups within the health and social care sector experience higher emotional exhaustion levels due to the nature of the individuals they serve and challenging working environments. Some of these groups include staff working in intensive care units,[26] child protection services,[27] hospice workers,[28] mental health professionals[29] and urology.[30] Their levels of compassion fatigue, burnout and psychological trauma increase more when their social support is limited, caseloads are high, and there is little autonomy to make work-related decisions.

More than 50 years ago, the first study into the emotional vulnerability of health professionals was published by Isabel Menzies. In her research, she looked at nurses who continuously cared exclusively for patients who had severe injuries or who were physically ill, and whose recovery was not always certain.[22] Many of the nurses dealt with suffering and death and found that caring for patients with incurable diseases was the most distressing part of their role. When caring for these patients, having physical contact (for example, washing their patients) stirred a range of powerful emotions in the nurses, from anxiety, love, pity and compassion, to worry, hatred and resentment. At the centre of these feelings was envy that the patients had such an abundant amount of care shown to them.

In an attempt to cope with the anxiety felt by the nurses, they depersonalized the patients and themselves, using a range of strategies:

- detachment and denial of their feelings;
- a task-list care system, absolving themselves from the anxiety associated with decision-making;
- referring to patients by the disease they had rather than by their name;
- nursing uniforms becoming a symbol of behavioural uniformity – there was no individualism; instead, one nurse was inter-changeable with another.

Evidence suggests that the experience of depersonalization of some healthcare staff relates to a difficulty in recognising negative emotions.[23] Furthermore, these healthcare staff can confuse negative emotions in patients, such as fear and anger, as positive ones. Not being able to sensitively understand those we support, and misinterpreting negative emotions as positive, has a significant impact. Expressions of sadness tend to prompt caring behaviours, and depersonalization is a factor contributing to this emotion being misread and not being responded to in certain cases.[24] Healthcare staff experiencing burnout may seek positive and rewarding signals in some patients while ignoring difficult emotions in others. It is unclear whether staff are aware of their misreading of these emotions and how they subsequently respond.

Despite health professionals experiencing high levels of burnout, including depersonalization, there is evidence suggesting that patients and independent observers often do not notice this this. So, despite feelings of significant burnout and higher levels of basal cortisol levels, physicians were able to maintain a professional approach. The effects of burnout appear to heighten in group GP practice environments compared with doctors working in their own single-handed practices.[25] A factor could be that group practices tend to place higher demands on staff, whereas single-handed GPs have more control and autonomy. To combat this, group practices can foster and support working environments where staff thrive, and the consequences of burnout would be buffered.

When to intervene

Some interventions support staff effectively to minimize the effects of burnout by managing their emotions and feelings of exhaustion and improving their job satisfaction. Professor Stefan DeHert, President of the European Society of Anaesthesiology, presented a simplified version of the development of burnout (Fig. 1 below).[31] I have used this to show indicators of when it might help intervene in order to halt burnout and prevent it from developing into a condition that severely hampers our physical and mental wellbeing. A caveat to this is that, as human beings, we are complex, as are our emotions, and we rarely 'fit' a model. However, it can help support our understanding of the processes we experience and how each stage affects the other stages.

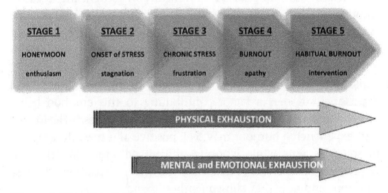

Figure 1 Simplified version of the development of burnout

Stage 1: Honeymoon

As previously discussed in Part I, students and newly qualified staff should receive training about ways to cope when working in health and social care systems that are emotionally and physically challenging. This potentially reduces the gap between the ideals they might hold about their job and what happens on the job in practice. They should expect to encounter stressors and know how to overcome these in order to avoid eroding their enthusiasm. We know that properly preparing staff for the job they will undertake, and the challenges associated with it, significantly reduces the risk of mental health problems.[32] Moral injury has been described by medical students who had found coping with working in prehospital and emergency care difficult, particularly when they were exposed to trauma that they felt they were not prepared for.[33] When helping professions aren't prepared for traumatic events, this potentially increases their fears. So, receiving training about what traumatic events might be experienced, expected psychological and behavioural responses, self-help strategies, and where to access appropriate resources could hugely prepare them for their careers.

Action

- **Preparation:** students and newly qualified staff are taught what to expect when working in challenging environments; events that might lead to trauma; the range of responses to this; and where to access support.
- **Prevention:** implement practices from Part I.

Stage 2 (onset of stress) and stage 3 (chronic stress)

This is the stage when the risks of burnout might be triggered as you experience more job-related stressors. It could be that you stop having boundaries, start working more overtime and start experiencing some days as more problematic than others. You might begin to feel more tense and irritable, and work might preoccupy you, even when you are not there. Sleep disturbances might start to happen, and family, friends and personal priorities might become neglected. Over time, this worsens, and you move into chronic stress. This stage is often characterized by a pervasive sense of powerlessness and feeling that the amount of effort you put in is not recognized, which then leads to feelings of inadequacy or incompetence.

Actions:

- Set boundaries (See 'Learning to say "No"' in Part I).
- If you have made plans with family or friends, try to stick to these.

- When away from work, try not to look at emails, take work calls, or respond to messages.
- Engage in activities and hobbies that help you feel relaxed, including exercise.
- Put strategies in place to help you to manage stress at work (see Chapter 13: The magic is in side you in Part I).
- Limit your alcohol and substance intake.
- Speak with someone you trust about how you are feeling.
- If you have a religious belief or spiritual practice, connect with this.
- Ensure you have adequate rest and sleep.
- Try some of the self-compassion and gratitude exercises in Part I.

Stage 4 (burnout) and stage 5 (habitual burnout)

When you feel enveloped in feelings of failure and power-lessness, this can create despair and disillusionment. You might experience apathy, and feel indifferent and cynical. The final stage is chronic burnout, and all of these symptoms will create physical and emotional exhaustion in you. Ideally, before reaching this stage, you will have shared how you have been feeling with someone.

Actions:

- **Seek professional support:** talking therapies from a therapist/ counsellor/psychologist.
- **Visit your GP:** some antidepressant medication has shown to be beneficial when used in combination with talking therapies.[34]

Substance use

When we start to use alcohol or other substances, no one can foresee the journey that lies ahead with it. Like others navigating complicated relationships with addiction, there are many reasons why health and social care staff also struggle. There is limited research into the prevalence and experiences of recovery for these staff groups. The available studies focus primarily on healthcare staff, and many of these are over 20 years old.

Like those with substance use and problem-related drinking in the wider population, there are many reasons why healthcare professionals might be at risk. Substance or alcohol use could be for practical reasons, such as trying to stay awake and alert on overnight or all-day shifts, or because of psychological motives – to manage the emotional pain arising from making difficult decisions and distressing work-related events. An increase in alcohol, caffeine and tobacco use is common following traumatic events. They can help users self-medicate distress or symptoms of traumatic stress. The development of substance or alcohol dependency often can't be linked to a single event. The complex interplay of personality, genetic predisposition, work-related stress, grief or an injury/accident at work, family stress, and co-morbid mental illness are risk factors for doctors to develop an addiction, and this is similar to the general population.[35]

Healthcare staff, particularly medical professionals, have knowledge of and access to different types of drugs. So, they might begin to use medications to manage pain, depression, anxiety or insomnia they have diagnosed and treat themselves. Health professionals have also reportedly used substances to manage stress and burnout due to working in health and social care.[36] Given the high prevalence of burnout and stress across these industries, relatively little is unknown about the prevalence and impact of drug and alcohol use on these groups. The focus has been primarily on physicians.

A survey reported that the prevalence of physician substance use was an 8 per cent lifetime rate of substance-use disorder, similar to the general American population.[37] Opiates and benzodiazepines were the only two kinds of prescription medications that physicians misused more than the general population. Using a sequential mixed-methods analysis examining the fitness to practice cases presented to the Nursing and Midwifery Council, in the UK, between 2014 and 2016, there were 208 alcohol-related cases and 131 cases of drug use brought forward.[38] Staff evidence also suggests that problematic substance use could be linked to occupational distress in paramedics.[39]

Drug- or alcohol-related problems don't occur overnight. They usually evolve over time, as this example illustrates:

Jane is an occupational therapist working in a forensic psychiatric unit. She enjoys her work and finds it fulfilling. Over the past couple of months, many staff have left to go to other jobs, and this has increased the pressure on Jane. When she returns home, it has become harder for her to unwind, and so she has started to have a glass of wine each evening. As time has gone on, she has found her mood becoming low and her alcohol intake in the evening increasing. As she drives home from work, it is all she can think about. Soon she is drinking a bottle of wine a night, and the following morning, not only does she feel ill, but she may also be over the driving limit. Jane knew her drinking was out of control but felt so embarrassed to ask for help. She went to the doctors to seek help with her mood and stress at work, and tried to manage her alcohol consumption herself.

For many helping professions, alcohol and some substance use can be used as a coping strategy to manage the demand of challenging work environments. This has been known to happen with social care as well as healthcare staff.[40] Many barriers stop us from reaching out for support often when we need it the most, which we discuss later.

Signs that you are developing or have developed a problematic relationship with substances or alcohol might include:[41]

- feeling that you have to use the substance regularly – daily or even several times a day;
- having intense urges for the substance that block out any other thoughts;
- over time, needing more of the substance to get the same effect;
- taking more significant amounts of the substance over a longer period than you intended;
- making sure that you maintain a supply of the substance;
- spending money on the substance, even though you can't afford it;
- not meeting obligations and work responsibilities or cutting back on social or recreational activities because of substance use;

- continuing to use the substance, even though you know it's causing problems in your life or causing you physical or psychological harm;
- failing in your attempts to stop using the substance;
- experiencing withdrawal symptoms when you attempt to stop taking the substance.

Recognizing signs of problematic substance or alcohol use in colleagues:[42]

- changing jobs frequently;
- preferring night shifts, when there is less supervision and more access to medication;
- falling asleep on the job or in-between shifts;
- volunteering often to administer narcotics to patients;
- anxiousness about working overtime or extra shifts;
- taking frequent bathroom breaks or unexplained absences;
- smelling of alcohol or excessively using breath mints or mouthwash;
- extreme financial, relationship or family stress;
- glassy eyes or small pupils;
- an unusually friendly relationship with doctors who prescribe medications;
- incomplete charting or repeated errors in paperwork.

As with others who use excessive drugs and alcohol, thoughts and attempts of suicide increase; this has also been reported in physicians.[43] Self-referrals into treatment programmes are not common. However, regulatory bodies, such as the General Medical Council in the UK, include a procedural track that allows substance misuse problems to be classed as a health problem. Rehabilitation and treatment are offered to support doctors to clinical practice, usually with extended supervision. Several organizations have been established to help healthcare professionals; some are listed in the Resources section at the end of this book.

16

Reaching out for support

I am reluctant to discuss the number of working days that are lost due to the compromised mental wellbeing of helping professionals, or the impact of this on service provision. While these are important considerations, they are positioned as a productivity and financial issue, rather than a need for systemic and organizational change where staff are nurtured and valued in their roles. We know staff continue to work despite experiencing mental health-related issues (presenteeism).[1]

When the helpers need helping, many struggle to reach out for support. And this is despite the workplace campaigns promoting the importance of mental wellbeing, the advice and support we offer to those we serve about seeking help, and possibly our jobs involving the promotion of reaching out for mental health support. Many factors contribute to staff feeling unable to admit to needing support, reaching out and receiving it.

As helping professions often wrapped within our professional (and even personal) identity, we are there to 'fix', solve, cure and ease others' suffering, which potentially heightens our sense of self-sufficiency. Also, the narrative many of us hold in our profession is to portray competence, as well as to instil confidence in those we support and care for. However, doing this minimizes our own needs and makes it difficult to seek help and take time off.[2]

Stigma

The perceived stigma that is associated with having compromised mental health in the helping profession is real. Many feel ostracized and don't disclose that they are struggling with issues relating to mental wellbeing. Evidence suggests that staff are reluctant to admit this to colleagues as it could negatively affect their career or their registering or licensing bodies could be alerted to the situation.[3] Helping professionals who have mental wellbeing issues are perceived to be unstable, less skilled in their role, and lacking in credibility. This might take the form of subtle or more overt messages from colleagues, leaders and the broader organization directed towards those who use mental health support or other help-seeking resources.

Additionally, we will have our own internal beliefs and perceptions of help-seeking, facilitating us to seek support or to avoid it. It's difficult to overcome our own hurdles, particularly when we don't recognize what these are. Many of you will have learned to consciously or subconsciously bury, hide from or run from your emotions. Between mental health symptoms beginning and staff seeking support, there is usually a considerable delay, which means many will have reached a crisis point before seeking support.[4] Tom, an occupational therapist, shares his experience of stigma in the workplace:

> I knew I had been feeling burnout for quite a few months. The service was under incredible strain, and we were all working hard to stay on top of things. I didn't notice it at first, the shift into becoming mentally unwell. An incident at work happened, and I thought I was managing it, but looking back now, it seems so obvious I wasn't. My sleep became more problematic. I struggled to feel happy about anything, and although I still turned up to work, my motivation was low. I started thinking maybe I didn't want to be here anymore. A good friend who I had cancelled meeting up with lots of times turned up at my door. He knew I wasn't myself. At first, I brushed it off, tried to change the conversation, but he persisted, and I'm glad he did. I shared with him how I was feeling, and he came with me when I spoke with my doctor. I took a few months away from work and got the support I needed.
>
> When I returned to my job, I felt pretty nervous, not sure how my colleagues would respond to me. Some were supportive, and others weren't. I would walk into a room, and they would stop talking, or I would hear them whispering when I left. I found out some colleagues would check my work without my knowledge to make sure I had done a good enough job. This continued, and a month later, I had lost a lot of confidence in my abilities. Their behaviours made me feel like I was incompetent and lacked credibility. I decided to leave that job. The

next one I went into, I was sure not to disclose my previous mental health struggles.

Tom's experience with his co-workers potentially stigmatizes him, influencing whether he reaches out for future support. It is therefore understandable that he might be silent in his next role in order to avoid discrimination and stigma.

The role silence plays in an organization when an individual is on mental-health-related sick leave and when they later return to work negatively impacts that individual and their colleagues. Social interactions at work can have a crucial part in either supporting our mental wellbeing or not. Many co-workers support the individual on sick leave if they are well liked and the symptoms relate to a specific stressful experience, so the silence is temporary.[5] In contrast, others' practices of silence can be punishing and dismissive.

Some workplace initiatives have been implemented to break down stigma and promote mental health and wellbeing, with significant success. This has involved helping professions sharing their personal experiences of mental illness.[6] Leadership and supervisor training programmes have also incorporated how these issues could be addressed with sensitive communication, the allocation of sufficient and supportive resources, and a commitment to facilitating cultural changes.[7, 8]

Shame and guilt

When staff reach out to me for support, they have often not disclosed to other colleagues, managers and sometimes family that they are seeking help. The reason is not just stigma but the shame they feel about needing support. When a client sees me for the first time, I haven't witnessed the hardship, conflict and turmoil they've possibly grappled with in deciding to seek input. However, over time it reveals itself: the struggle many professionals face in overcoming the barriers to reach out for support.

At the core of moral injury are feelings of shame and guilt. Even in the absence of moral injury or distress, the thread of shame is usually in the narrative of many experiences:

- 'I can't just get on with it.'
- 'All my colleagues seem to be coping better than me.'
- 'Is there a reason why I'm so affected by the multiple deaths I've seen during the COVID-19 crisis?'
- 'I don't deserve help.'
- 'I think there's something wrong with me.'

The list of these could be endless. When the hook of shame becomes embedded in us, we can be completely debilitated by it. We might not even be aware that it is shame we are feeling, so our behaviours can also be good indicators that we are not ourselves. Shame might show up as:[9]

- physically withdrawing, silencing ourselves, and keeping secrets;
- pleasing others and seeking to appease;
- trying to gain power by aggression or shaming and blaming others.

Brené Brown discusses that being human means that we won't be able to avoid shame. However, we can experience it without compromising our identity and values, which she calls 'shame resilience'. In developing this, the first step is to recognize how shame shows up in you: anger, withdrawal, blaming others. The second step is identifying what has triggered it, and, lastly, acknowledging that shame disconnects us from others. So, when we have empathy and compassion for ourselves and others, shame struggles to mutate.

As helping professionals, many decisions we make will be ethical and heart-driven, rather than rational reasoning. This is because we are human, and we bring our whole selves to the work we do. That might have a cost, in that we are emotionally wounded at times by the very things we love or did love: our jobs. Noticing how shame shows up in our bodies, in our minds and in our behaviour is an important step.

Exercise: Feeling shame

Recall a situation or decision you made or didn't make, or an inter-action with a colleague, where you felt shame.

What was it about that experience that left you feeling shame?

_____

_____

_____

What judgement does your mind make about you? (For example, 'You're stupid', 'You're weak.')

_____

_____

_____

What did you feel in your body?

_____

_____

_____

If you had a similar experience in the future, how might you show more empathy and self-compassion?

_____

_____

_____

17

Reaching in to support others

Imagine this scenario for a moment: a colleague whom you see most days shows up. They have been badly beaten up. Their face and body are covered in bruises, they limp when they walk, and they don't mention what everyone else can see. Many staff rally around with enquiries about what has happened, how they feel, and the need to take time away from work, reassuring them that their workload will be covered.

Now imagine this scenario: a colleague whom you see most days shows up. They are a little bit quiet, but they carry on with their work. You are busy, so you don't take any more notice until three weeks later when they turn up looking unkempt. You ask if they are okay, and they say, 'Yes, I'm fine.' Again, as the weeks pass, they look more tired, but it is a busy time at work, and everyone is feeling the strain. Two months later, when you arrive at work, they aren't there, and your manager shares that they are off on sick leave. When you meet up for a coffee with them away from work, they share the months of mental turmoil and distress they have been suffering, following a serious case review they were involved in, which identified them as having missed numerous opportunities to intervene.

In the first scenario, the suffering is evident and relatable because we all know what it's like to feel physical pain. Also, we expect a physical assault to affect someone, so we are cued socially to respond to this with empathy and compassion. In the second scenario, the pain and suffering are less noticeable. How people behave doesn't necessarily match what they're feeling on the inside, so it requires us to tune into the subtle and more obvious mental distress signs. However, the fundamental difference between the first and second scenarios is expectation. When working in emotionally challenging environments where traumatic and adverse events are experienced, we don't always expect our colleagues to be psychologically affected. In the first scenario, space was created, giving the person 'permission' to feel. In the second, there were fewer opportunities. This is not necessarily to assume that everyone wants to talk or is negatively affected by serious events. Instead, it's about creating an opportunity for support if somebody wants it. Many of us address one another with 'Morning, how are you?' – but is that a greeting, or is it an invitation to say: *I'm here, I'm making the space, and I have time to listen to whatever you give me right now.* If colleagues want to talk, you need to be prepared to listen.

Not everyone who experiences adverse events will have a trauma response: we all process experiences differently. For some of you, just knowing there is someone there can be enough to help you feel safe and better able to cope. Therefore, the culture of psychological safety within the organization, the role of leadership, and the range of support offered become crucial in supporting those who require it.

Early interventions

Everyone working in health and social care organizations should receive mental health literacy training, irrespective of their position, role or pay grade. Mental health literacy involves many elements,[1] including recognizing different types of psychological distress, specific disorders, and knowledge and beliefs about interventions available.

An increase in knowledge doesn't necessarily result in reducing workplace stigma or unhelpful attitudes. Rather than imparting generic information, this training should be tailored to specific contexts, so everyone is better able to recognize signs day-to-day. This would mean that when our colleagues' mental wellbeing is identified, we are better able to know what the tipping point for action is.

Early interventions have shown to be effective in supporting helping professionals experiencing mental distress and trauma. Psychological first aid (PFA)[2] is one such intervention that aims to reduce the initial distress caused by traumatic events by developing short- and long-term coping. There could be several staff within the team or organization trained in PFA and can be accessed when needed.

There are five principles of PFA:

1 *Promoting safety: removing individuals from immediately traumatic experiences and protecting them from secondary trauma.* For helping professionals, this would mean that after a potentially traumatic event which resulted in serious injury or fatality – for example, being assaulted at work, or involved in care that did not go as expected – staff involved would be able to go home and not be expected to remain in work.

2 *Calming: reducing arousal symptoms can be achieved through relaxation techniques and providing information about assessing and managing their traumatic experience.* At these times, grounding techniques (see Part I – Grounding) can help them feel less overwhelmed and actively help them shift attention away from their thoughts and back to the outside world.

3 *Increasing self-efficacy: identifying internal and external ways to reduce the stress reactions and take a proactive role in their trauma recovery.* This might include supporting staff to reconnect with the ways they have been able to manage difficult situations in the past. For example, this could be through walking, listening, connecting with nature, or journaling how they feel. It would also entail reinforcing the need for rest and to eat and look after themselves.

4 *Connection: supporting staff to connect with existing social support systems and, if helpful, ways to build additional supportive networks with colleagues, mentors, supervisors and others external to work.* This might involve making a list with the person about the people they have in their life they feel safe and relaxed with and those who provide practical and professional support to them.

5 *Hope and optimism: helping individuals see they won't always feel this way.* Although, at the moment, retaining information might be compromised, reassuring staff that people recover from distressing and traumatic events will be of help.

Leadership and psychological safety

Support from colleagues and line managers will play an instrumental part in safeguarding staff mental health.[3] If you are in a senior or in a leadership position, you have a significant role in the prevention of and response to your workforce's trauma, which requires you to actively reach out and connect with those you are there to serve (staff).

Taking an active approach and reaching out to staff following traumatic events is crucial in reducing their distress. Avoidance is a key symptom of trauma that can leave individuals feeling isolated and frightened. You should pay particular attention to those staff who cancel meetings and are too busy and unreachable. For these staff and those who have been psychologically affected, the suggestion of support from you might be appreciated. By prioritizing offers of support to staff, where they feel listened to, with empathy and understanding, particularly in the initial phase following the event, you will help their distress and promote recovery.[4]

Staff will be highly tuned to your behaviours as a leader. So, when traumatic events happen, many staff will look to you for reassurance and guidance, and clear communication is essential, especially at these times. At the time of writing, the death toll from COVID-19 continues to grow. The loss of life, both personally and professionally, is beyond what many helping professions have ever encountered. Alongside caring for loved ones with COVID-19, many staff have also cared for and treated colleagues who have sadly died. As well as feelings of trauma, compassion fatigue, burnout and moral injury, large swathes of staff are grieving significant losses. This grief and loss need addressing.

Leaders of organizations will need to voice what has been lost and support staff to find a way through. This will involve providing hope about the future and the recovery while acknowledging that the pandemic continues, and that if it does end, then there will still be issues and challenges, as there were pre-COVID-19. Leaders will need to connect with the organization's values and demonstrate integrity, and ensure that what they say aligns with what they do. And they must show that their desire to support staff is measurable; for example, by securing funding for a range of mental health support and letting staff know that they are able to access these programmes during work hours. One-off interventions will not suffice and can cause additional harm.[5] Indeed, one-off interventions can unhelpfully convey the message to staff that their distress and trauma-related feelings will be resolved in a single session. Leaders should also remember that they are human too; recognizing their own reactions to distress and implementing or seeking support are critical to ensure that their own wellbeing is also optimized.

Being able to normalize staff reactions will feel emotionally containing for many while promoting and drawing on the staff group's strength to enable to support one another if they feel able to. Having psychologically safe teams will be particularly advantageous in facilitating this.

A psychologically safe culture is one where all team members feel supported rather than scrutinized, where they feel seen and heard, and where attention is paid to what is communicated and how it is communicated.[6] A leader's behaviour is critical in creating psychologically safe cultures. Team members will feel psychologically safer when they are led democratically and supportively, and encouraged to question and challenge. By contrast, leaders who are defensive and authoritarian will leave staff feeling less able to speak out because their team is unsafe.

Creating emotional and psychological safety for staff experiencing trauma is crucial in the progress of their recovery. Amy Edmondson, a professor at Harvard Business School, first identified the concept of psychological safety in teams, following her work researching staff in hospitals. Here is a checklist she created. You can use this to reflect on the level of psychological safety in your team.

Exercise: Your team's psychological safety

Use the following checklist to reflect on the safety of the team you currently work in:

- I can make a mistake on this team and it will usually not be held against me.
- I can safely take risks on my team.
- On my team, those who are different are accepted.
- I trust that my teammates would not deliberately undermine my efforts.
- My unique skills and talents are valued and utilized when I work with my teammates.
- I can readily ask my teammates for help.
- My teammates and I can bring up problems and tough issues.

If you answer 'yes' to all the questions above, then you are probably working in a team with high levels of psychological safety.

Routine support

After experiencing trauma, it is not uncommon for you to feel as though your sense of safety has been compromised or reduced. This can feel very frightening and can heighten your sense of vulnerability. In response to these feelings, you might have a strong desire to hide away, even from those who know and love you the most. Although isolating from others and restricting your activities might feel protective, it reduces the access you have to helpful social support networks.[7]

Social connection positively benefits those experiencing psychological distress. However, when shame and guilt, which are core symptoms of moral injury, are central to that distress, many people want to withdraw. Having routine support that staff can access regularly will normalize the need to seek the support for themselves when working in challenging roles and will optimize their mental wellbeing. Additionally, it will help them learn from and create meaningful narratives from their experiences, rather than traumatic ones, when trauma has occurred. Healing often begins in a moment of connection with another, which routine support can serve. Here are some evidence-based supports that effectively provide ongoing psychological support to others and when they experience traumatic events.

Peer-to-peer programmes

As discussed, there are many barriers to staff reaching out and seeking support. Peer support programmes are not there to replace mental health professional input. Instead, staff can find it easier to speak with peers who have had similar experiences to their colleagues and are trained in offering support and signposting resources and services. Peer support services are not just there for those who are experiencing trauma or mental health difficulties. They are also designed to support colleagues experiencing any work-related stressors or personal challenges. Speaking with others within your industry, who understand the issues you are facing, can help intervene before you feel your mental wellbeing is significantly compromised. They can also break the stigma of reaching out for support and offer the comfort of knowing you are not alone.

Schwartz rounds

Schwartz rounds provide a space for clinical and non-clinical staff to reflect on their work's emotional challenges. This emphasizes connecting with colleagues' experiences rather than the technical aspects of their role, thus enabling a more inclusive discussion. Meetings are usually held every four to six weeks and last for 60 minutes approximately. Evaluation of their efficacy has indicated that they positively impact the psychological wellbeing of staff, who report feeling less stressed and alone in their experience, fostering a greater sense of cohesiveness.[8] Staff report feeling more focused on demonstrating their values of compassion and kindness, better understanding their colleagues' experiences, and having greater appreciation for them.[9]

Clinical supervision

For helping professions, clinical supervision is the lynchpin with which we continue to develop our self-awareness, knowledge, abilities and skills. It gives us a safe space to explore the emotional impact of the roles we hold. Clinical supervision doesn't replace learning and additional training but should serve to enhance them. Concerns can be raised in supervision, which can then help prevent issues escalating and our emotions from reaching crisis points. Here is a helpful framework that categorises the functions of clinical supervision:[10]

- **Normative:** this includes reviewing, maintaining, and developing care standards concerning safety, ethics, and quality practice.
- **Formative:** developing professional knowledge and skills enables helping professions to incorporate reflection and its application into practice.
- **Restorative:** self-development and self-awareness abilities are enhanced. The value of clinical supervision for health and social care staff is widely recognized, with some staff groups incorporating this into their practice more than others. Change and challenging times are inevitable within helping professions, and clinical supervision can provide a supportive forum to develop and flourish.

Group restorative supervision

The uptake of individual clinical supervision within some organizations has been hampered by funding restrictions or insufficient cover for staff to attend. It is accepted that many staff groups need a space where they can share, develop and connect with others. Therefore, restorative group supervision has been offered to support professionals working within emotionally challenging environments. Studies evaluating the effectiveness of group supervision have found it positively benefits those involved. Not only did it reduce the effects of stress and burnout on staff, but it also had additional benefits.[11]

1 **Facilitating insight:** staff have reported being able to have a more comprehensive understanding of the wider impact of their individual style on their team and have been supported to make changes.
2 **Helping deal with conflicts:** the space created within group supervision is psychologically safe. Therefore, where conflict has happened within the group, supervision has provided an opportunity to support staff to manage it and to also draw on the group to demonstrate how factors might worsen the situation or mediate it.
3 **Normalizing:** understanding how colleagues feel and how this might be similar to you has a powerful impact in normalizing the feelings and responses of working in emotionally challenging environments. It also provides opportunities for staff to hear how others cope with these.
4 **Fostering creativity:** bringing together staff with different ideas can create innovation and support rethinking new ways to approach situations or incorporate different practices within services.

Group supervision can help optimize staff mental wellbeing, normalize the effects of working in challenging environments bring, and foster a sense of innovation and team cohesion.

Exercise: Your support mechanisms

What support can you access regularly? (weekly, fortnightly, monthly)

_____

_____

_____

If you can't access this in your organization, is there a group you and your colleagues could create? (virtual or in-person)

_____

_____

_____

What might you need to support the creation of this? (practical, emotional, organizational)

_____

_____

_____

Are there groups outside your organization you can access? If so, what are they?

_____

_____

_____

What steps do you need to take to enable you to reach out to this support?

_____

_____

_____

_____

18
It's good to talk

There are many evidence-based psychological therapies for the treatment of trauma-related symptoms and PTSD in adults. All of these trauma-focused treatments involve you connecting with the traumatic event and are summarized in this chapter.

Eye movement desensitization and reprocessing (EMDR) therapy[1]

What is it?

EMDR is an individual therapy usually delivered across six to twelve sessions, once or twice a week. It requires you to connect directly with the trauma memory. It does not include extended exposure to the trauma memory, detailed descriptions of the stressing memory, challenging trauma-related beliefs, or homework assignments.

It involves eight phases:

- Phase 1: History-taking
- Phase 2: Preparing the client
- Phase 3: Assessing the target memory
- Phases 4–7: Processing the memory to an adaptive resolution
- Phase 8: Evaluating treatment results.

How does it work?

This approach has been informed by the adaptive information processing model. This holds that PTSD symptoms continue to cause distress because the memory of the disturbing historical experiences has not been processed sufficiently. It is believed that the emotions, beliefs, thoughts and physical sensations experienced during the traumatic event are contained within these unprocessed memories. Unlike other treatments for PTSD, EMDR therapy focuses directly on the memory by altering how the memory is stored in the brain, thereby minimizing and eradicating the trauma-related symptoms.

The procedures that EMDR uses, such as eye movements, taps and tones while the individual focuses on the trauma memory, simultaneously reduce the memory's intensity and emotion by accelerating, it is believed, the learning process.

Cognitive behavioural therapies

Cognitive behaviour therapy (CBT) has been used in the treatment of PTSD, and three additional interventions derived from CBT are designed especially to support those impacted by traumatic experiences: cognitive processing therapy, cognitive therapy, and prolonged exposure.

Cognitive processing therapy (CPT)[2]

CPT is usually delivered over 12 sessions and teaches you how to modify and challenge unhelpful beliefs developed about the trauma. By learning this, you create a new understanding of the traumatic event, which reduces the associated symptoms and minimizes their effects on your life.

Cognitive therapy (CT)[3]

CT is usually delivered, either individually or in groups, weekly over three months. The cognitive model for PTSD suggests that you will develop PTSD if you process a traumatic event that has led to you experiencing severe threat at that moment. This is due to the negative appraisals of the trauma and your subsequent feelings and thoughts or because of how your memory of the trauma has been processed. Consequently, unhelpful coping strategies are developed in an attempt to manage the associated negative cognitions and emotions. CT treatment aims to alter the appraisals and memories so as to disrupt the thoughts and behaviours that are negatively affecting your life.

Prolonged exposure (PE)[4]

Like many CBT approaches, PE is usually provided over three months, with weekly sessions lasting between one and two hours. It has the largest evidence-base supporting its efficacy in the treatment of PTSD.

When you have experienced trauma, it is understandable that many will want to avoid any reminders of the trauma, as this serves to reinforce the associated fear. PE attempts to support you to learn to approach the memories, feelings and situations associated with the trauma. Doing so reduces PTSD symptoms because you learn that the trauma-related memories and triggers aren't dangerous, so they don't need to be avoided.

Given how critical safety supports are to those who are impacted by trauma, the therapeutic relationship is essential to create such supports before commencing PE. Two types of exposure are used, imaginal and in vivo, and you, not the therapist, lead the pace of this.

- **Imaginal exposure:** this occurs in the session with you describing the traumatic event, using the present tense.
- **In vivo exposure:** this involves tackling the fear stimuli away from the therapy room and also homework assignments.

Some studies suggest that up to 60 per cent of helping professionals will benefit from exposure therapy. This means that a considerable number would require a different type of support.[5] Other therapies have been recommended where there is evidence that they can lead to positive outcomes. These therapies aren't included in treatment recommendations and guidelines because the evidence might not be as strong or not as relevant for subgroups of PTSD presentations and treatment settings. However, additional research could strengthen the evidence for using them, and they could be recommended in future guidelines.

Acceptance and commitment therapy (ACT, said as one word)[6]

CT is a behavioural treatment, and central to it is the idea that suffering doesn't come from the emotional pain we feel but our attempts to avoid that pain. It accepts that human suffering is inevitable, so the overall goal is to enhance psychological flexibility, be present in the moment, accept difficult internal experiences, and live a life of meaning (values).

Although ACT has been used to treat a range of other mental health conditions, there is expanding evidence for the benefit of using ACT to treat PTSD.

How does it work?

ACT holds that we usually have low psychological flexibility levels when we experience PTSD because our behaviour is dominated by avoiding trauma-related stimuli and internal experiences (thoughts, feelings, sensations, memories). This is achieved through the following processes:

- *Recognizing that trying to escape from emotional pain won't work (called creative hopelessness).* You engage in therapy activities that provide you with insight into all of the ways you've been trying to avoid emotional pain (e.g. drinking excessively, withdrawing from friends, getting a different job) but which haven't worked to remove the pain you're experiencing.
- *Learning that control is the problem, not the solution.* ACT holds that it is in the attempt to avoid or control emotional pain that the problems lie. So, by spending time trying to avoid or control how you feel, there's little energy left to pursue the things in life that are important to you (e.g. relationships), worsening your emotional pain.
- *You are not your thoughts.* We've discussed earlier in this book that thoughts can feel very strong, and we can interpret them as facts. After a traumatic event, your mind might start to tell you that you're 'damaged', 'unlovable' or a 'bad person'. You learn how to become an observer of your thoughts, take a step back from them, and not get hooked on them.
- *Stop struggling.* You are taught ways to let go of your attempts to avoid or control thoughts and feelings, and practise being willing and open to experience them as they are, not how your mind tells you they are.

- *Committed action.* Values, that is, the areas of your life that are important, are identified and you are supported to demonstrate behaviours that reflect them while being willing to feel or observe the thoughts that might arise as a result.

Somatic therapy[7]

Rather than focusing only on thoughts or emotions associated with the traumatic event, somatic therapy incorporates the natural bodily (somatic) responses to the trauma.

How does it work?

Dr Peter A. Levine developed this therapy in the 1970s. He observed that, after animals had recovered from repeated traumatic experiences (attempted attacks by predators) and the threat was gone, the animal continued to release their fight-or-flight energy physically by shaking, trembling or running. When they had completed their physical release, they were then able to return to their normal state. Dr Levine believes that after we experience traumatic events, we try to 'keep it together, and in doing so, our natural release cycle is hampered'. Consequently, this perpetuates the state of fight-or-flight, and so we are unable to return to a state of balance and relaxation.

In somatic therapy, you don't necessarily examine the memories or emotions associated with a traumatic event but uncover the bodily sensations linked to those feelings.

Finding a therapist

What to ask?

Many therapists will often offer a 15 to 30- minute free consultation. Finding the right person with whom you feel safe and connected, and a good 'fit', is essential in supporting you on your healing journey. I think it's helpful to meet a few different therapists before deciding with whom to begin this work. I would suggest not getting into the details of the traumatic event, as this might not be psychologically safe for you. Rather, write down generally what happened, the impact it's having on your life, and what in your life you want to support. For example, 'I encountered a traumatic event at work. Since then, I've tried to manage it, but I'm finding I'm having problems sleeping, I get pretty anxious when I go to work, and I don't feel I'm coping well. I would like some support to begin to work through this experience and start to feel better.'

All therapists will be registered with a professional organization and you can check out who might be available in your area. Below are some questions you can ask them and some questions you might want to reflect on after meeting them.

Exercise: Assessing a potential therapist

Questions to ask a potential therapist
1. How long have you been practising?
2. What licences and certifications do you have, and which professional organizations do you belong to?
3. How many clients have you worked with similar difficulties to me?
4. How much do you charge? (Also, whether there are options for sliding scale.)
5. What happens to our work together when you go on annual leave?

Reflections after meeting a potential therapist
1. How emotionally and physically safe did I feel?
2. Do I feel like I could trust this person?
3. Did I feel connected with them, that we had a good rapport?
4. Was our conversation awkward or uncomfortable?
5. Did I feel comfortable in their office?
6. Did they ask me good questions?
7. Did they seem knowledgeable, confident and skilled?
8. Did I want to leave quickly, or could I have stayed longer?
9. Did I feel seen, understood and listened to?
10. How would I feel about seeing them again?
11. How was my body while I was speaking with them?
12. What is my gut instinct saying about this therapist?

Pharmacotherapy

People experiencing PTSD aren't routinely offered medication. However, if you have depression, sleep problems (caused by PTSD), or are unable to access talking therapies, medication might be provided, prescribed by your GP or a mental health specialist such as a psychiatrist. They include:

- paroxetine
- mirtazapine
- amitriptyline
- phenelzine
- venlafaxine
- sertraline.

Depending on your symptom severity, personal history, side effects, co-morbidities and response to these medications, other medications might be prescribed.

Most of your working environments are physically and emotionally challenging at times. Being part of caring and safe teams and having access to routine support to reflect on these challenges and connect with one another will help you feel secure in your team. Being able to *reach out* for help and *reach in* to colleagues when they need it the most will reflect the psychologically safe culture you're working in, which means you will be met with openness and compassion, rather than discrimination and prejudice. If you have experienced a traumatic event at work, this will be fundamental in optimizing your mental wellbeing. In increasingly overstretched services, routine support is desperately needed, as is being able to access specialist help if you require this, without feeling guilt and pressure from your team and organization when you take time away from work to engage in this. These necessitate the mental wellbeing of safety and the provision of quality of care provided to patients, service users or clients.

Sleep

Most people will have sleep-related issues at some time over their career. However, after a traumatic experience, sleep disturbances are common – the quantity and quality of your sleep changes.[8] You might have trouble falling asleep, wakefulness during sleep, or early-morning insomnia. This is because, after a traumatic event, your body will be experiencing a stress response, displaying the symptoms of hyperarousal (such as feeling jumpy) and being hyper-alert. This contributes to insomnia. Some evidence suggests that trauma can affect how our body moves through the sleep stages and cycles. Rapid eye movement (REM) sleep, which processes emotions and stores memories, is believed to be most affected.[9]

Distressing dreams or nightmares are also common and returning to sleep after these can be difficult. These dreams might contain trauma-related symbols, content and emotions, whereas the nightmares might be directly related to the traumatic event itself. It is believed this is due to the brain's fear response, coupled with hyperarousal, and could be our mind's way of trying to make sense of the event.[10]

Being able to sleep after a traumatic event can support the healing process. Some research indicates that targeting sleep issues soon after experiencing trauma could reduce the risk of developing PTSD.[11] Furthermore, being able to sleep has also been shown to reduce trauma-related memories, making them less distressing.[12]

While implementing effective sleep hygiene will significantly support your healing following a traumatic event, being able to have good sleep habits, independent of trauma, will benefit your mental wellbeing. If you are receiving support from a therapist, psychologist or psychiatrist, they too can help you with achieving realistic sleep goals during your recovery.

Tips for good sleep hygiene

- *Sleep where you feel safe:* often after a traumatic event we don't feel safe, making it tricky to fall asleep. Think through where you might feel safest sleeping. You might want someone sleeping next to you.
- *Try to avoid alcohol, coffee and other substances:* stimulants will exacerbate symptoms of hyperarousal and alertness, which will interfere with sleep.
- *Establish a bedroom routine:* having a predictable routine before bed can also create feelings of safety. Engaging in a relaxing activity can support your body's natural relaxation response, supporting you to feel calmer before bed.
- *Maintain your typical sleep pattern:* if your work schedule has changed, try to establish a sleep routine, when you go to sleep and get up at the same time. This can support you having quality sleep. If you feel tired during the day, try to rest, rather than nap.
- *Get up:* it might sound counterintuitive but because our brain makes associations quickly, if you're awake in bed, tossing and turning, it might begin to associate bed with wakefulness. If after 20 minutes you're still awake, it might be better to get out of bed and either read or listen to some gentle music, keeping the lights dim. Avoid looking at screens if possible.

19
Final words

It has been estimated that almost 90 per cent of the population will be exposed to at least one traumatic event during their lifetime[1] but that fewer than 10 per cent will go on to develop PTSD.[2] Most people who experience PTSD or trauma-related symptoms make a full recovery. As Dr Peter Levine has shared, 'Trauma is a fact of life. It does not, however, have to be a life sentence.' Everyone processes trauma in their own way and at their own pace, and most people recover from it.

Working in challenging environments can be emotionally difficult for many helping professionals. Our bodies do a great job of letting us know that we have been affected by an event, situation or interaction. They're not the only indicator. Our behaviours can also shed some light on our internal landscape. Being able to listen and observe these and connecting with ourselves is crucial.

Expect to have an emotional or physical response when you experience difficult circumstances at work. Some people experience a work-related traumatic event or a series of events that accumulate and that will render them physically and psychologically unwell. Again, this is your brain and body's way of trying to make sense of something that has profoundly affected you.

Self-care, in isolation, isn't a magic cure to prevent the effects of trauma, burnout, compassion fatigue or moral injury. Many other factors will contribute to giving you the best chance to be mentally healthy during your career. Teaching the next generation of helping professionals about the realities of the profession, ways to prevent themselves from becoming unwell, and optimizing their mental wellbeing will massively equip them when they are inevitably faced with the challenges they encounter at work.

Changing our behaviour is tough, and forming healthier habits is more complicated than just having the proper knowledge and an abundance of willpower. Knowing why it's important to us to take better care of ourselves can help with our motivation. Being able to set goals that are small, achievable and measurable will also be necessary. Minor, incremental changes can make a massive difference over time. However, this effort can be redundant if we don't have the support systems (practical and emotional) to enable us to practise and maintain the change. In the case of behaviour change, being forewarned is definitely forearmed. Setting If–Then plans can help us to acknowledge the situations that make it difficult for us to change our behaviour and the ways we can overcome these situations. Therefore, a combination of goal setting, support and If–Then plans can enhance the likelihood of us achieving the goal and maintaining the changed behaviour.

You bring your whole self to work, and learning ways to protect yourself when you're in your role will support you and those you are caring for. When we know what we stand for in life, connect with our values, and reflect on these behaviours, we can feel more confident and fulfilled. However, having this clarity, particularly about work-related values, while it can be helpful, can also be wounding when the organization is set up so that the valued actions are suffocated. Observing our thoughts and fostering self-compassion in the face of these situations will potentially mitigate the impact this distress can create.

Practising self-compassion is a way for you to have a relationship with yourself (and others) that is nurturing, respectful and empathetic. When I hear and witness staff being unkind, judgemental and insensitive to colleagues or those they support in their role, I can see this as a symptom. To hold our needs, or those of another, in mind, we need to make space for that in our heads and hearts. This is difficult to do when we are overstretched, disrespected or not valued by the organization. Disconnection, therefore, becomes a necessity to survive in a workplace that is harmful to us.

Just as our feelings and behaviours can indicate how we might be feeling, toxic workplaces can also be viewed as a wounded organization. Vicarious trauma, compassion fatigue, moral injury and burnout experienced by some of our most exhausted colleagues impact on all who come into contact with them. This impact varies to a lesser or greater degree when we ruminate on how colleagues' rude behaviours affect us. Not only does it dilute the care staff provide, as well as subsequent interactions, but it can erode our mental wellbeing. Leaders play an instrumental role in stamping these behaviours out and creating environments where they are not allowed to develop. Acts of kindness benefit everyone, the giver and the receiver, so we mustn't underestimate their power. We don't have to feel infused with feelings of kindness to be kind. However, we need to have a mindset and know which actions to practise daily that demonstrate kindness in our jobs.

Being positive and having a positive mindset doesn't mean accepting these behaviours or putting up with workplaces that harm us, but it can help us work better within them. Working in health and social care will be stressful at some points, and this is to be expected. However, juggling multiple stressors, perhaps on a daily basis, is corrosive to our mental wellbeing. If we surround ourselves with positive influences that can significantly boost our mental health, we can better cope under stress and connect more with ourselves and others. Being faced with multiple daily stressors not only impacts us psychologically, but it affects us physically. Many situations, like being alone, having too many responsibilities, or working in a challenging environment, can overwhelm the ventral vagus system. Being aware of that and practising ways to tone your vagus nerve, preferably daily, will optimize your body's chances of managing stressful situations better.

Part of your trauma experience will be that you have some arousal symptoms, such as being easily startled, tense, or feeling 'on-guard'. Sleep is critical in reducing these symptoms. The majority of those experiencing trauma will likely have some degree of disturbed sleep. Developing healthy sleeping habits in the absence of trauma will undoubtedly be advantageous, should you encounter sleep difficulties at any time in your career. Seeking additional support from your medical provider can also be helpful when experiencing trauma-related sleep disturbances.

We are not emotional islands; instead, we are social beings. However, trauma-related feelings or distress where shame is a pervasive feature might result in us withdrawing or isolating ourselves from others at times when we most need support. In the journey to seeking support, you might engage in behaviours that contribute to the distress you're experiencing. To ask for help is an act of courage. It is a choice to turn towards that part of you that is emotionally hurting and hold it with the care and love it so undoubtedly deserves.

Staff need to feel safe to feel. Many decisions you make won't always be based on rational reasoning. Instead, they're driven by your heart. Of course they will be, because, for many, your passion, love and desire to improve the lives of those suffering have been the drivers for you to enter your chosen profession. Instead of the organization and team reinforcing the need to repress your emotions, safe spaces must be created and resources developed to normalize the challenging environments you work in. This requires courageous leaders to model the behaviour they want in their organizations. Working in psychologically safe environments won't eradicate experiences of adversity. However, it can significantly buffer the effects traumatic events might have. Again, leaders play an instrumental part in this.

As our world becomes faster-paced and technology advances, we are losing sight of the humans in health and social care. The responsibility of leaders is to keep the staff they serve at the centre of the organisation. In your leadership role, modelling behaviours and talking about the impact of events will support your workforce. By communicating with empathy and transparency, and creating spaces for staff to share their experiences without fear of retribution, will help them make meaning of the event(s). However, you too need to attend to your own feelings and reactions to distress and likewise care for yourself in such a way that you can be fulfilled as a leader.

The COVID-19 pandemic has had a remarkable effect on health and social care staff. Many of you have had to, and will continue to, navigate through unchartered territories in your role while battling with the workload, lack of resources, and the added threat of ill health to you, your colleagues and your loved ones. Some of these strains will undeniably have been present before the pandemic. They will likely have become exacerbated, and many of you will be negatively affected psychologically. However, at each level, there are many opportunities to influence your mental wellbeing positively, find meaning in the events that happened, and create growth opportunities. We might work in buildings, rely on technology, and have an abundance of policies and procedures in place, but people make up 'the system', and it's the connection with others that is the foundation of human care. Protecting the system and those in it with nurture, compassion and care is critical to optimizing the mental wellbeing of the staff who undoubtedly have earned it.

As professionals working in health and social care, whether you're in the infancy of your career or have years of experience, change is possible. You can love your job and be healthy in body and mind. It might be that you picked up this book to start that journey, or you want to strengthen some of the practices you already implement in your life. Whatever the reason, I hope you have found something here that speaks to you, but more importantly, you have learned that recovery is possible, and that you are very deserving of it.

Appendix: Exercises

Exercise
Creating new habits
What is my goal?
Why is it important for me to pursue this goal?
When will I start my goal?
When will I practise it?
What needs to be in place before I begin pursuing my goal?

Barriers	
Internal (thoughts, feelings, etc.)	*External* (environment, situational)

If–Then Plan	
Step 1 (If): Situations	*Step 2 (Then): Solutions*

Which supportive person(s) can I share my goal with?
What are the signs to me I am benefitting from this goal?
How will I reward myself when I have reached it?
What date will I review how effective it is?
What changes (if any) do I need to make?

Exercise: Defining your emotions

Take a recent situation where you experienced a strong emotion and try to connect with the feelings you felt at the time.

What were the broader emotions you were feeling (hurt, sadness, happiness, anger)?

_____

_____

Now, try to connect with the emotion that might be under that? (You can use the table above as a prompt to help you.)

_____

_____

_____

Exercise: What does vulnerability mean to you?

Many of us have a complicated relationship with the word 'vulnerable', so let's start by thinking about what it means to you.

Write down all the words that come to mind when you think of the word 'vulnerable'.

_____

_____

_____

This exercise is adapted from Brené Brown's work in *Daring Greatly*. Think of **three** examples where you recently felt vulnerable, then answer the following questions for each one

Name the situation – for example, *in work.*

_____

_____

_____

What was the circumstance or trigger? *I couldn't input something into the computer system.*

_____

_____

_____

How did you feel? *I felt stupid and incompetent.*

_____

_____

_____

How might you react if you were daring greatly (i.e., using courage and willingness to engage with those around you)? *Admit I don't know how to do it and ask a colleague for help.*

_____

_____

Exercise: Connecting how you feel in your body

- Take a moment, breathe in deeply, and exhale fully.
- **How** is my body feeling right now?

_____

_____

- **Where** in my body am I feeling _____?
- **What** is the feeling I am experiencing?

_____

_____

- If this (area of my body) could speak right now, what would it say?

_____

_____

- Take a moment, breathe in deeply, and exhale fully.

Exercises: Grounding techniques

The 5-4-3-2-1 grounding technique

This technique uses all five senses to support you to try to get back to the present moment. You can do this sitting down or standing up.

- Take a couple of deep breaths, breathing in fully and out fully. Look around you and aloud, or in your mind, name:

  five things you can see in the room you're in or outside the window

  four things you can feel – it could be the texture of your clothing, an object in front of you, a slight breeze on your skin...

  three things you can hear (birds outside, ticking of your clock, traffic, people talking)

  two things you can smell

  one thing you can taste.

- Finally, a couple of deep breaths, breathing in fully and out fully.

Colour

- Choose a colour, any colour; it doesn't matter.
- How many different shades of that colour can you see in the room you are in or out of the window?
- Choose another colour, and repeat until you notice your feelings beginning to ease.

Counting

Start at 100, and count backwards by 6. This usually requires a lot of concentration.

Others

- Listen to your favourite music.
- Go for a walk.
- Move your body: stretching, dancing, running up and down stairs. Due to the adrenalin pumping through our bodies when we are in this cycle, some people find movement helps displace some of this energy. They are then better prepared to do more calming grounding techniques.

Exercise: Creating your work-related values

- Write a sentence to summarize your valued direction. For example, *I want to be a caring, attentive and patient nurse.*

_____

- Rate out of 10 how important this value is to you – where 0 = *low importance* and 10 = *high importance.*

    Low 0 1 2 3 4 5 6 7 8 9 10 High

- Rate how successfully you have lived this value during the past month on a scale of 0 (*not at all successfully*) to 10 (*very successfully*).

    Not at all 0 1 2 3 4 5 6 7 8 9 10 Very

- What behaviours might reflect this is your value, for example acts of kindness to patients and colleagues (the more you can list, the better).

_____

_____

_____

Barriers are inevitable, and considering these in advance can help you to think about ways to overcome them when they arise. What might get in the way of you demonstrating this value? Write one or two words to remind you of the barriers you will face to pursue your valued path and strategies to help you accept them.

Barriers	Strategies
Feeling stressed	Take a moment – breathe. Do the 5-4-3-2-1 grounding technique. Tell myself: 'This will pass.'

Exercise: When are you judgemental?

To have greater insight into when your mind might be more critical and judgemental, write down the times you notice this happening and how you respond.

Events, situations or circumstances when I feel critical:
for example, *when I have made a mistake at work.*

_____

What does my mind say?
You're foolish for doing that – can't you get anything right?

_____

How I could respond with patience and kindness?
I was in a rush, I'm tired, and I was trying my best. Next time, I need to give myself a little more time.

_____

Exercise: Self-compassion break

This exercise can be applied in the moment and takes only a few minutes.

Bring to mind a situation in your life that is causing you upset or some stress (not the most extreme one).

How does this situation make you feel? Where in your body do you feel the emotion? When you feel connected to the situation and associated feelings, try saying the following affirmations to yourself, either out loud or in your mind:

- 'This hurts' or 'I'm finding this stressful' – this will activate mindfulness.
- 'All of us sometimes suffer in life', 'I am not alone', 'others feel this way, too' – remember common humanity and that part of being human means we will suffer at some point; it is unavoidable.
- 'I will try to be kind to myself', 'May I be patient with myself' or 'I will forgive myself' – whatever you think is most appropriate for your situation.

Exercise: Best friend voice

Being self-compassionate involves recognizing that being imperfect and failing is inevitable, and that life will have its difficulties. However, resisting this as reality can result in feeling self-critical and often stressed. Learning to accept this with kindness and gentleness can move us closer to a more self-compassionate space.

I like this exercise below as it can help us see when our mind is being unkind to us and our inner critic is being loud. It encourages us to consider how we would treat others if they were in that situation versus how we treat ourselves. If you feel able to, it might be helpful to write down your answers to this.

- Bring to mind a time when you struggled at work. It might have been something you got wrong, a situation which didn't go as planned, or the way you behaved with a colleague or someone you were helping.
- Next, what did your mind say to you about this? Did it make judgements about you? Was it bullying you? Were the criticisms loud? What tone does this take? What are you feeling? Where in your body were you feeling it?
- Now think about a friend or a loved one coming to you. When you have that image in your mind, read out your situation, thoughts and feelings as if it were their experience.
- Imagine how you would feel when they shared this with you and your response. How would your tone be? What might you say?
- If you feel able to, write this down. Take a moment and read this through, connecting with the words and sentiment.
- Next, think about how you could use this when you're in a similar situation in the future. You might write out just a few words or a sentence to guide you at that moment to mindfully enhance your self-compassion.

Exercise: Challenging your inner critic

What has happened?
For example, *spoke rudely to a colleague.*

_____

What did you notice your inner critic said?
You're a horrible person.

_____

How did this make you feel?
Guilty, like a bad person.

_____

_____

What words of understanding and compassion could you say in
response?
*You were tired and in a rush. You're not a mean person. Go to your
colleague and apologize for what you said.*

_____

_____

Exercise: Learning to say 'no'

When do you notice you find it difficult to be assertive at work?

_____

_____

What does your mind say and your body feel during these interactions?

_____

_____

If you struggle to say 'no', what else could you say or do?

_____

_____

When might you try this out?

_____

_____

What might get in the way of you doing this?

_____

_____

_____

_____

Exercise: Coping with feelings

Use the following questions as a guide to support you as you think about how you feel when feelings arise at work that you find difficult to manage, how you might respond to these, and what you might do differently.

What situations, people, or events trigger emotions you find difficult to cope with at work?

_____

_____

_____

_____

_____

What does your mind say and your body feel?

_____

_____

_____

_____

How could you respond in a way that is kind to yourself?

_____

_____

_____

_____

_____

Exercise: Random acts of kindness

List the random acts of kindness you could action:

_____

_____

_____

_____

_____

Over the next four weeks, list some of the acts of kindness you can show to:

Yourself:

_____

_____

_____

Colleagues:

_____

_____

_____

Loved ones:

_____

_____

_____

Exercise: Connecting with your autonomic states

Recall memories that might help you connect with the three states and write a few sentences or words to help you recognize signs when you shift into each of them.

- **Collapse or shutdown** (dorsal states can sometimes feel numb, floppy or foggy)

_____

_____

- **Fight or flight** (sympathetic states might feel energixing and charged)

_____

_____

- **Safe and connected** (ventral vagal states might feel calm, passionate, joyful)

_____

_____

Exercise: Using anchors

When you're activated and are heading towards fight/flight or shutdown mode, anchors are a great way to draw you back to your ventral vagal state and help you stay there. With regular practice, anchors can strengthen your ability to manage difficult emotions, using who, what, where and when categories. Try to write as many examples as you can.

- **Who?** Make a list of the people (and the pets) in your life who make you feel safe and content when you're with them. This list could also include those who are no longer alive or are spiritual beings.

  _____

  _____

  _____

- **What?** Think about things you do that make you feel alive, nourished or joyful. It could be something simple like watering your plants or going for a walk. Again, think of the micro-moments that you feel grateful for.

  _____

  _____

  _____

- **Where?** These are the places where you feel connected and safe. It could be somewhere in your home, community, neighbourhood, or a place you can access at work.

  _____

  _____

  _____

- **When?** Recollect the memories when you felt safe. It could be moments or more extended periods.

  _____

  _____

  _____

Exercise: Are you practising defensively?

What are subtle and obvious signs that you might be practising defensively?

Subtle signs: _____

_____

Obvious signs: _____

_____

Recall a time when your actions were defensive. What were you feeling at that time?

_____

_____

Rather than the action you took, what could you have done to manage the emotions you were experiencing?

_____

_____

What other actions could you have taken, rather than defensive?

_____

_____

What do you need in place to practise less defensively?

_____

_____

If this is not possible currently, are there alternative ways to support yourself?

_____

_____

Exercise: Feeling shame

Recall a situation or decision you made or didn't make, or an inter-action with a colleague, where you felt shame.

What was it about that experience that left you feeling shame?

_____

_____

_____

What judgement does your mind make about you? (For example, 'You're stupid', 'You're weak.')

_____

_____

_____

What did you feel in your body?

_____

_____

_____

If you had a similar experience in the future, how might you show more empathy and self-compassion?

_____

_____

_____

Exercise: Your team's psychological safety

Use the following checklist to reflect on the safety of the team you currently work in:

- I can make a mistake on this team and it will usually not be held against me.
- I can safely take risks on my team.
- On my team, those who are different are accepted.
- I trust that my teammates would not deliberately undermine my efforts.
- My unique skills and talents are valued and utilized when I work with my teammates.
- I can readily ask my teammates for help.
- My teammates and I can bring up problems and tough issues.

If you answer 'yes' to all the questions above, then you are probably working in a team with high levels of psychological safety.

Exercise: Your support mechanisms

What support can you access regularly? (weekly, fortnightly, monthly)

_____

_____

_____

If you can't access this in your organization, is there a group you and your colleagues could create? (virtual or in-person)

_____

_____

_____

What might you need to support the creation of this? (practical, emotional, organizational)

_____

_____

_____

Are there groups outside your organization you can access? If so, what are they?

_____

_____

_____

What steps do you need to take to enable you to reach out to this support?

_____

_____

_____

_____

Exercise: Assessing a potential therapist

Questions to ask a potential therapist

1. How long have you been practising?
2. What licences and certifications do you have, and which professional organizations do you belong to?
3. How many clients have you worked with similar difficulties to me?
4. How much do you charge? (Also, whether there are options for sliding scale.)
5. What happens to our work together when you go on annual leave?

Reflections after meeting a potential therapist

1. How emotionally and physically safe did I feel?
2. Do I feel like I could trust this person?
3. Did I feel connected with them, that we had a good rapport?
4. Was our conversation awkward or uncomfortable?
5. Did I feel comfortable in their office?
6. Did they ask me good questions?
7. Did they seem knowledgeable, confident and skilled?
8. Did I want to leave quickly, or could I have stayed longer?
9. Did I feel seen, understood and listened to?
10. How would I feel about seeing them again?
11. How was my body while I was speaking with them?
12. What is my gut instinct saying about this therapist?

References

1 The cost of caring for helpers

1. Figley, C.R. (ed.) (1995). *Compassion Fatigue: Coping with Secondary Traumatic Stress Disorder in Those Who Treat the Traumatized*. New York: Brunner/Mazel, p. 1.
2. World Health Organization. Burn-out an 'occupational phenomenon': International Classification of Diseases. Available at: www.who.int/mental_health/evidence/burn-out/en/
3. Reith, T.P. (2018). Burnout in United States healthcare professionals: a narrative review. *Cureus* 10(12): e3681. doi:10.7759/cureus.3681
4. Jameton, A. (1984). *Nursing Practice: The Ethical Issues*. Englewood Cliffs, NJ: Prentice-Hall.
5. Litz, B.T., Stein, N., Delaney, E., Lebowitz, L., Nash, W.P., Silva, C., et al. (2009). Moral injury and moral repair in war veterans: a preliminary model an intervention strategy. *Clinical Psychology Review* 29, 695–706.
6. Greenberg, N., Docherty, M, Gnanapragasam. S., and Wessely S. Managing mental health challenges faced by healthcare workers during COVID-19 pandemic. *BMJ*, 368: m1211.
7. Smith, J. (2021). *Nurturing Maternity Staff: How to Tackle Trauma, Stress and Burnout to Create a Positive Working Culture in the NHS*. London: Pinter & Martin, 2021.

2 Trauma responses

1. Morganstein, J.C., West, J.C., and Ursano, R.J. *Work-Associated Trauma. In (2019). Work Associated Trauma*. In M.B. Riba, S. Parikh and J. Greden (eds), *Mental Health in the Workplace: Strategies and Tools to Optimize Outcomes*. Cham, Switzerland: Springer Nature Publishing Company.

4 The wonder nerve

1. Laborde, S., Mosley, E. and Thayer, J.F. (2017), Heart rate variability and cardiac vagal tone in psychophysiological research: Recommendations for experiment, planning, data analysis, and data reporting. *Frontiers in Psychology* 8:213. doi: 10.3389/fpsyg.2017.00213.

2. Maran, T., Sachse, P., Martini, M., and Furtner, M. (2017). Benefits of a hungry mind: When hungry, exposure to food facilitates proactive interference resolution. *Appetite* 108, 343–52. doi: 10.1016/j.appet.2016.10.023

5 Prevalence of work-related adversity

1. Beck, C.T. (2011). Secondary traumatic stress in nurses: A systematic review. *Archives of Psychiatric Nursing* 25(1): 1–10.
2. Hunter, B., Fenwick, J., Sidebotham, M., and Henley, J. (2019). Midwives in the United Kingdom: Levels of burnout, depression, anxiety and stress and associated predictors. *Midwifery* 79.
3. Hunter., B, Henley, J., Fenwick, J. et al. (2018). *Work, Health and Emotional Lives of Midwives in the United Kingdom: The UK WHELM Study*. School of Healthcare Sciences, Cardiff University.
4. Caringi, J.C., Hardiman, E.R., Weldon, P., Fletcher, S., Devlin, M., and Stanick, C. (2017). Secondary traumatic stress and licensed clinical social workers. *Traumatology* 23(2): 186–95.
5. Beyond Blue (2019). *National Mental Health Survey of Doctors and Medical Students*. Australia.
6. Baugerud, G.A., Vangbaek, S., and Melinder, A. (2018). Secondary traumatic stress, burnout and compassion satisfaction among Norwegian child protection workers: protective and risk factors, *The British Journal of Social Work* 48(2): 215–35.
7. Maunder, R.G., Lancee, W.J., Balderson, K.E., Bennett, J.P., Borgundvaag, B., Evans, S., Fernandes, C.M., Goldbloom, D.S., Gupta, M., Hunter, J.J., McGillis Hall, L., Nagle, L.M., Pain, C., Peczeniuk, S.S., Raymond, G., Read, N., Rourke, S.B., Steinberg, R.J., Stewart, T.E., VanDeVelde-Coke, S., … Wasylenki, D.A. (2006). Long-term psychological and occupational effects of providing hospital healthcare during SARS outbreak. *Emerging Infectious Diseases* 12(12): 1924–32.
8. Cottler, L.B., Ajinkya, S., Merlo, L.J., Nixon, S.J., Abdallah, A.B., and Gold, M.S. (2013) Lifetime psychiatric and substance use disorders among impaired physicians in physicians' health program: Comparison to a general treatment population. *Journal of Addiction Medicine* 7(2): 108–12.
9. Greenberg, N., Weston, D., Hall, C., Caulfield, T., Williamson, V., Fong K. (2020). The mental health of staff working in intensive care during COVID-19. Available from: www.medrxiv.org/content/10.1101/2020.11.03.20208322v2.
10. Beck, C.T. (2011). Secondary traumatic stress in nurses: A systematic review. *Archives of Psychiatric Nursing* 25(1): 1–10.

11. Hunsaker, S., Chen, H.C., Maughan, D., and Heaston, S. (2015). Factors that influence the development of compassion fatigue, burnout, and compassion satisfaction in emergency department nurses. *Journal of Nursing Scholarship* 47(2): 186–94.
12. Peckham, C. (2018). *Medscape National Physician Burnout and Depression Report 2018*. Available from: www.medscape.com/slideshow/2018-lifestyleburnoutdepression-6009235.

6 Building a foundation

1. Michie, S., van Stralen, M.M., and West, R. (2011). The behaviour change wheel: a new method for characterising and designing behaviour change interventions. *Implementation Science* 6(1).
2. Neal, D.T., Wood, W., and Quinn, J.M. (2011). Habits: A repeat performance. *Current Directions in Psychological Science* 15(4): 198–202.
3. Coats, E.J., Janoff-Bulman, R., and Alpert, N. (1996). Approach versus avoidance goals: Differences in self-evaluation and wellbeing. *Personality and Social Psychology Bulletin* 22: 1057–67.
4. Elliot, A.J., and Thrash, T.M. (2002). Approach-avoidance motivation in personality: approach and avoidance temperaments and goals. *Journal of Personality and Social Psychology* 82: 804–18.
5. Gollwitzer, P.M., and Sheeran, P. (2006). Implementation Intentions and Goal Achievement: A meta-analysis of effects and processes. In M.P. Zanna (ed.), *Advances in Experimental Social Psychology* (pp. 69–119). San Diego, CA: Elsevier Academic Press.
6. Locke, E.A., and Latham, G.P. (2006). New directions in goal-setting theory. *Current Directions in Psychological Science* 15(5): 265–8.

8 Who are you?

1. Smith, J. (2021). *Nurturing Maternity Staff: How to Tackle Trauma, Stress and Burnout to Create a Positive Working Culture in the NHS*. London: Pinter & Martin, 2021.

10 Fostering self-compassion

1. Neff, K.D., and Pommier, E. (2012). The relationship between self-compassion and other-focused concern among college undergraduates. *Self and Identity*, 1–17. doi:10.1080/15298868.2011.649546
2. Rockliff, H., Gilbert, P., McEwan, K., Lightman, S., and Glover, D. (2008). A pilot exploration of heart rate variability and salivary cortisol responses to compassion-focused imagery. *Clinical Neuropsychiatry* 5.

3. Gustin, L.W., and Wagner, L. (2013). The butterfly effect of caring: Clinical nursing teachers' understanding of self-compassion as a source to compassionate care. *Scandinavian Journal of Caring Sciences* 27: 175–83.
4. Gilbert, P. (2009). *The Compassionate Mind: A New Approach to the Challenges of Life*. London: Constable & Robinson.
5. Neff, K. D. (2003). Self-compassion: An alternative conceptualization of a healthy attitude toward oneself. *Self and Identity* 2, 85–102.
6. Gilbert, P., and Irons, C. (2005). Focused therapies and compassionate mind training for shame and self-attacking. In P. Gilbert (ed.), *Compassion: Conceptualisations, Research and Use in Psychotherapy* (pp. 263–325). London: Routledge.
7. Barnard, L.K., and Curry, J.F. (2011). Self-compassion: Conceptualizations, correlates, and interventions. *Review of General Psychology* 15(4): 289–303.
8. Kabat-Zinn, J. (1982). An outpatient program in behavioral medicine for chronic pain patients based on the practice of mindfulness meditation: theoretical considerations and preliminary results. Retrieved from: www.ncbi.nlm.nih.gov/pubmed/7042457
9. Raab, K. (2014). Mindfulness, self-compassion, and empathy among health care professionals: A review of the literature. *Journal of Health Care Chaplaincy* 20(3): 95–108.

11 Navigating toxic workplaces

1. Taştan, S.B. (2017). Toxic workplace environment: In search for the toxic behaviours in organizations with a research in healthcare sector. *Postmodern Openings* 8(1): 83–109.
2. Bowling, N.A., Alarcon, G.M., Bragg, C.B., and Hartman, M.J. (2015). A meta-analytic examination of the potential correlates and consequences of workload. *Work & Stress* 29: 95–113.
3. Heyworth, J. (2004). Stress: A badge of honour in the emergency department? *Emergency Medicine Australasia* 16: 5–6.
4. Potter, C. (2006). To what extent do nurses and physicians working within the emergency department experience burnout: A review of the literature. *Australasian Emergency Nursing Journal*, 9: 57–64.
5. Global strategy on human resources for health: Workforce 2030 – World Health Organization, 2016.
6. Duffy, E. (1995). Horizontal violence: A conundrum for nursing. *Journal of the Royal College of Nursing* 2(2): 5–17.
7. McKenna, B.G., Smith, N.A., Poole, S.J., and Coverdale, J.H. (2003). Horizontal violence: Experiences of registered nurses in their first year of practice. *Journal of Advanced Nursing* 42(1), 90–6.

8. Hunter, B., Henley, J., Fenwick, J. et al. (2018). *Work, Health and Emotional Lives of Midwives in the United Kingdom: The UK WHELM Study*. School of healthcare Sciences, Cardiff University.

9. The Royal College of Midwives (RCM), *Evidence to the NHS Pay Review Body* (2017) [Online]. Available from: www.rcm.org.uk/media/1911/rcm-evidence-nhs-pay-review-2017.pdf [Accessed 28/02/21]

10. Bureau of Labor Statistics. (2014). *Occupational Outlook Handbook: Social Workers*. Retrieved from Rishel, C.W., Hartnett, H.P., and Davis, B.L. (2016). Preparing students to provide integrated behavioral health services in rural communities: The importance of relationships in knowledge-building and practice. *Advances in Social Work* 17: 151–65

11. Ibid.

12 Unlocking the power of positivity

1. Fredrickson, B.L., Mancuso, R.A., et al. (2000). The undoing effect of positive emotions. *Motivation and Emotion* 24, 237–58.

2. Fredrickson, B.L., and Levenson, R.W. (1998). Positive emotions speed recovery from the cardiovascular sequelae of negative emotions. *Cognition and Emotion* 12: 191–220.

3. Emmons, R., McCullough, M. (2003). Counting blessings versus burdens: An experimental investigation of gratitude and subjective wellbeing in daily life. *Journal of Personality and Social Psychology* 84(2): 377–89.

4. Buchanan, K., and Bardi, A. (2010). Acts of kindness and acts of novelty affect life satisfaction. *Journal of Social Psychology* 150(3): 235–7.

5. Zahn R., Garrido G., Moll J., and Grafman J. (2014). Individual differences in posterior cortical volume correlate with proneness to pride and gratitude. *Social Cognitive and Affective Neuroscience* 9, 1676–83

6. Moll, J., Krueger, F., Zahn, R., Pardini, M., de Oliveira-Souza, R., and Grafman, J. (2006). Human fronto-mesolimbic networks guide decisions about charitable donation. *Proceedings of the National Academy of Sciences USA* 103: 15623–8.

7. McCraty, R., Barrios-Choplin, B., Rozman, D., Atkinson, M., and Watkins, A.D. (1998). The impact of a new emotional self-management program on stress, emotions, heart rate variability, DHEA and cortisol. *Integrative Physiological and Behavioral Science* 33(2): 151–70.

8. Emmons, R. (2013). *Gratitude Works!: A 21–Day Program for Creating Emotional Prosperity*. Hoboken, NJ: Wiley.

9. Zahn, R. et al. (2009). The neural basis of human social values: evidence from functional MRI. *Cerebral Cortex* 19: 276–83.

13 The magic is inside you

1. Porges, S.W. (2010). Music therapy and trauma: Insights from the polyvagal theory. In Stewart, K. (ed.), *Symposium on Music Therapy and Trauma: Bridging Theory and Clinical Practice*. New York: Satchnote Press.
2. Kharrazian, D. (2013). *Why Isn't My Brain Working? A Revolutionary Understanding of Brain Decline and Effective Strategies to Recover Your Brain's Health*. Battle, UK: Elephant Press.
3. Greene, C.M., Craft Morgan, J., Traywick, L.S., and Mingo, C.A. (2017). Evaluation of a laughter-based exercise program on health and self-efficacy for exercise, *The Gerontologist* 57(6): 1051–61.

15 Behaviours as symptoms

1. Castel, E.S., Ginsburg, L.R., Zaheer, S., et al. (2015). Understanding nurses' and physicians' fear of repercussions for reporting errors: clinician characteristics, organization demographics, or leadership factors? *BMC Health Services Research* 15: 326.
2. Garcia-Retamero, R., and Galesic, M. (2014). On defensive decision making: How doctors make decisions for their patients. *Health Expectations* 17: 664–9.
3. Kachalia, A., Gandhi, T.K., Puopolo, A.L., Yoon, C., Thomas, E.J., Griffey, R., Brennan T.A., and Studdert, D.M. (2007). Missed and delayed diagnoses in the emergency department: a study of closed malpractice claims from 4 liability insurers. *Annals of Emergency Medicine* 49: 196–205.
4. Hoffman, J.R., and Kanzaria, H.K. (2014). Intolerance of error and culture of blame drive medical excess. *BMJ* 349: g5702.
5. Panella, M., Rinaldi, C., Leigheb, F., et al. (2017). Prevalence and costs of defensive medicine: a national survey of Italian physicians. *Journal of Health Services Research & Policy* 22: 211–7.
6. Bourne, T., Wynants, L., Peters, M., et al. (2015). The impact of complaints procedures on the welfare, health and clinical practise of 7926 doctors in the UK: A cross-sectional survey. *BMJ Open* 5: e006687.
7. Blendon, R.J., DesRoches, C.M., Brodie, M., Benson, J.M., Rosen, A.B., Schneider, E., et al. Views of practicing physicians and the public on medical errors. *The New England Journal of Medicine* 347(24): 1933–40.
8. Gallagher, T.H., Waterman, A.D., Ebers, A.G., Fraser, V.J., and Levinson, W. (2003). Patients' and physicians' attitudes regarding the disclosure of medical errors. *JAMA* 289(8): 1001–7.
9. Rowin, E.J., Lucier, D., Pauker, S.G., Kumar, S., Chen, J., and Salem, D.N. (2008). Does error and adverse event reporting by physicians and nurses differ? *The Joint Commission Journal on Quality and Patient Safety* 34(9): 537–45.

10. Wild, D., Bradley, E.H. (2005). The gap between nurses and residents in a community hospital's error-reporting system. *The Joint Commission Journal on Quality and Patient Safety* 31(1): 13–20.

11. Jeffe, D.B., Dunagan, W.C., Garbutt, J., Burroughs, T.E., Gallagher, T.H., Hill, P.R., et al. (2004). Using focus groups to understand physicians' and nurses' perspectives on error reporting in hospitals. *The Joint Commission Journal on Quality and Patient Safety* 30(9): 471–9.

12. Elwyn, G., Coulter, A., Laitner, S., Walker, E., Watson, P., and Thomson, R. (2010). Implementing shared decision making in the NHS. *BMJ* 341: c5146.

13. Spatz, E.S., Krumholz, H.M., and Moulton, B.W. (2017). Prime time for shared decision making. *JAMA* 317: 1309–10.

14. Vento, S, Cainelli, F., and Vallone, A. (2018). Defensive medicine: It is time to finally slow down an epidemic. *World Journal of Clinical Cases* 6(11): 406–9

15. Harris, N. (1987). Defensive social work. *British Journal of Social Work* 17(1): 61–9.

16. Jones, R. (2014). *The Story of Baby P: Setting the Record Straight*, Bristol, Policy Press.

17. Munro, E. (2004). The impact of audit on social work practice, *British Journal of Social Work* 34(8): 1075–95.

18. Munro, E. (2010). *The Munro Review of Child Protection: Part One: A Systems Analysis*. London, The Stationery Office.

19. Parton, N., and O'Byrne, P. (2000) *Constructive Social Work: Towards a New Practice*. Basingstoke, Palgrave Macmillan.

20. Webb, S.A. (2006) *Social Work in a Risk Society*. Basingstoke, Palgrave Macmillan.

21. Hughes, P., Brandenburgh, N., Baldwin, D.J., et al. (1992). Prevalence of substance use among US physicians. *JAMA* 267(17): 2333–9.

22. Menzies, I. (1960). A case study in the functioning of social systems as a defence against anxiety. *Human Relations* 13: 95–121.

23. Colonnello, V., Carnevali, L., Russo, P.M., Ottaviani, C., Cremonini, V., Venturi, E., and Mattarozzi, K. (2021). Reduced recognition of facial emotional expressions in global burnout and burnout depersonalization in healthcare providers. *PeerJ* 9: e10610

24. Seidel, E.-M., Habel, U., Kirschner, M., Gur, R.C., and Derntl, B. (2010). The impact of facial emotional expressions on behavioral tendencies in women and men. *Journal of Experimental Psychology: Human Perception and Performance* 36(2): 500–7.

25. Orton, P., Orton, C., and Pereira Gray, D. (2012). Depersonalised doctors: a cross-sectional study of 564 doctors, 760 consultations and 1876 patient reports in UK general practice. *BMJ Open 2*: e000274.

26. Pastores, S.M., Kvetan, V., Coopersmith, C.M., et al. (2019). Workforce, workload, and burnout among intensivists and advanced practice providers: A narrative review. *Critical Care Medicine* 47: 550–7.

27. Kim, H. (2011). Job conditions, unmet expectations, and burnout in public child welfare workers: How different from other social workers? *Children and Youth Services Review* 33(2), 358–67.

28. Quinn-Lee, L., Olson-McBride, L., and Unterberger, A. (2014). Burnout and death anxiety in hospice social workers. *Journal of Social Work in End-of-Life & Palliative Care* 10(3): 219–39.

29. Morse, G., Salyers, M.P., Rollins, A. L., Monroe-DeVita, and M. Pfahler, C. (2012). Burnout in mental health services: A review of the problem and its remediation. *Administration and Policy in Mental Health and Mental Health Services Research* 39: 341–52.

30. *Medscape National Physician Burnout & Suicide Report 2020*. Available from: www.medscape.com/slideshow/2020-lifestyleburnout6012460

31. De Hert, S. (2020). Burnout in healthcare workers: Prevalence, impact and preventative strategies. *Local and Regional Anesthesia* (28)13: 171–83.

32. Iversen, A.C., Fear, N.T., Ehlers, A., et al. (2008). Risk factors for posttraumatic stress disorder among UK armed forces personnel. *Psychological Medicine* 38: 511–22.

33. Murray, E., Krah., C., and Goodsman, D. (2018). Are medical students in prehospital care at risk of moral injury? *Emergency Medicine Journal* 35: 590–4.

34. Kaschka, W.P., Korczak, D., and Broich, K. (2011). Burnout: A fashionable diagnosis. *Deutsches Ärzteblatt International* 108: 781–7.

35. Brooks, D., Edwards, G., and Andrews, T. (1993). Doctors and substance misuse: Types of doctors, types of problems. *Addiction* 88: 655–63.

36. Windover, A.K., Martinez, K., Mercer, M.B., Neuendorf, K., Boissy, A., and Rothberg, M.B. (2018). Correlates and outcomes of physician burnout within a large academic medical center. *JAMA Internaal Medicinel*, 178(6): 856–8. Available from: https://jamanetwork.com/journals/jamainternalmedicine/fullarticle/2672575

37. Monroe, T.B., Kenaga, H., Dietrich, M.S., Carter, M.A., and Cowan, R.L. (2013). The prevalence of employed nurses identified or enrolled in substance use monitoring programs. *Nursing Research* 62, 10–15.

38. Searle, R., Rice, C., McConnell, A., and Dawson, J. (2017). Bad apples? Bad barrels? Or bad cellars? Antecedents and processes of professional misconduct in UK health and care, research paper. Professional Standards Authority of Health and Social Care. Available from: www.professionalstandards.org.uk/docs/default-source/publications/antecedent-amp-processes-of-professional-misconduct-in-uk-health-and-social-care.pdf?sfvrsn=1e087320_0

39. Hichisson, A.D., and Corkery, J.M. (2020). Alcohol/substance use and occupational/post-traumatic stress in paramedics. *Journal of Paramedic Practice* 12(10): 388–96.

40. Guhan, R., and Liebling-Kalifani, H. (2011). The experiences of staff working with refugees and asylum seekers in the United Kingdom: A grounded theory exploration. *Journal of Immigrant & Refugee Studies* 9, 205–28.

41. Mayo Clinic. https://www.mayoclinic.org/diseases-conditions/drugaddiction/symptoms-causes. Retrieved on 06/04/21.

42. Addiction Centre. https://www.addictioncenter.com/addiction/medical-professionals. Retrieved on 06/04/21.

43. British Medical Association (1993) *The Morbidity and Mortality of the Medical Profession*. British Medical Association, London.

16 Reaching out for support

1. Rosvold, E O., and Bjertness, E. (2001). Physicians who do not take sick leave: Hazardous heroes? *Scandinavian Journal of Public Health* 29(1), 71–75.

2. Harris, L.M., Cumming, S.R., and Campbell, A.J. (2006). Stress and psychological well-being among allied health professionals. *Journal of Allied Health* 35(4): 198–207.

3. Wallace, J.E., Lemaire, J.B., and Ghali, W.A. (2009). Physician wellness: A missing quality indicator. *The Lancet* 374: 1714–21.

4. Moll, S.E. (2014). The web of silence: A qualitative case study of early intervention and support for healthcare workers with mental ill-health. *BMC Public Health* 8(14): 138.

5. Hyman, I. (2008). *Self-Disclosure and Its Impact on Individuals Who Receive Mental Health Services*. Rockville, MD: Center for Mental Health Services, Substance Abuse and Mental Health Services Administration.

6. Kitchener, B.A, and Jorm, A.F. (2004). Mental health first aid training in a workplace setting: a randomized controlled trial. *BMC Psychiatry* 4(1): 23.

7. Gilbert, M., and Bilsker, D. (2012). *Psychological Health and Safety: An Action Guide for Employers*. Canada: Mental Health Commission of Canada and the Centre for Applied Research in Mental Health & Addiction.

8. Brown, B (2012). *Daring Greatly: How the Courage to be Vulnerable Transforms the Way We Live, Love, Parent and Lead*. New York: Gotham Books, p. 77.

9. Ibid.

17 Reaching in to support others

1. Jorm A.F. (2000). Mental health literacy public knowledge and beliefs about mental disorders. *British Journal of Psychiatry* 177(5): 396–4011.
2. Nusbaum, K.E., Wenzel, J.G., and Everly, G.S. (2007). Psychologic first aid and veterinarians in rural communities undergoing livestock depopulation. *Journal of the American Veterinary Medical Association* 231: 692–4.
3. Greenberg, N., Thomas, S., Iversen, A., Unwin, C., and Hull, L., (2003). Who do military peacekeepers want to talk about their experiences? Perceived psychological support of UK military peacekeepers on return from deployment. *Journal of Mental Health* 12, 565–73.
4. Brewin, C.R., Andrews, B., and Valentine, J.D. (2000). Meta-analysis of risk factors for posttraumatic stress disorder in trauma-exposed adults. *Journal of Consulting and Clinical Psychology* 68(5): 748–66.
5. Brooks, S.K., Rubin, G.J., and Greenberg, N. (2019). Traumatic stress within disaster-exposed occupations: overview of the literature and suggestions for the management of traumatic stress in the workplace. *British Medical Bulletin* 129: 25–34.
6. Edmondson, A. (1999). Psychological safety and learning behavior in work teams. *Administrative Science Quarterly* 44(2): 350–83.
7. Rubin, G.J., Brewin, C.R., Greenberg, N., Simpson, J., and Wessely, S. (2005). Psychological and behavioural reactions to the bombings in London on 7 July 2005: Cross-sectional survey of a representative sample of Londoners. *BMJ* 331(7517): 606.
8. Deppoliti, D. I., C.t.-Arsenault, D., Myers, G., Barry, J., Randolph, C., Tanner, B. (2015). Evaluating Schwartz Center Rounds® in an urban hospital center. *Journal of Health Organization and Management* 29(7), 973–987
9. Chadwick, R., Muncer, S. J., Hannon, B., Goodrich, J., and Cornwell, J. (2016). Support for compassionate care: Quantitative and qualitative evaluation of Schwartz Center Rounds in an acute general hospital. *Journal of the Royal Society of Medicine Open* 7(7).
10. Cassedy, P. *First Steps in Clinical Supervision*. Berkshire: Open University Press, 2010.
11. Wallbank, S. (2013). Maintaining professional resilience through group restorative supervision. *Community Practice* 86(8): 26–8.

18 It's good to talk

1. Shapiro, F. (2017). *Eye Movement Desensitization and Reprocessing (EMDR) Therapy: Basic Principles, Protocols and Procedures*, 3rd edn. New York, NY: Guilford Press.

2. Resick, P.A., Monson, C.M., and Chard, K.M. *Cognitive Processing Therapy for PTSD: A Comprehensive Guide*. A Guilford Press publication.

3. Ehlers, A., Hackmann, A., Grey, N, Wild, J., Liness, S., Albert, I., and Clark, D.M. (2014). A randomized controlled trial of 7-day intensive and standard weekly cognitive therapy for PTSD and emotion-focused supportive therapy. *American Journal of Psychiatry* 171: 294–304

4. Hembree, E.A., Rauch, S.A.M., and Foa, E.B. (2003). Beyond the manual: The insider's guide to prolonged exposure therapy for PTSD. *Cognitive and Behavioral Practice* 10(1): 22–30.

5. Hagenaars, M.A., van Minnen, A., and Hoogduin, K.A.L. (2010). The impact of dissociation and depression on the efficacy of prolonged exposure treatment for PTSD. *Behaviour Research and Therapy* 48(1): 19–27.

6. Thompson, B.L., Luoma, J.B., and LeJeune, J.T. (2013). Using acceptance and commitment therapy to guide exposure-based interventions for posttraumatic stress disorder. *Journal of Contemporary Psychotherapy* 43, 133–40.

7. Levine, P. (1997). *Waking the Tiger: Healing Trauma*. North Atlantic Books.

8. Babson, K.A., and Feldner, M.T. (2010). Temporal relations between sleep problems and both traumatic event exposure and PTSD: a critical review of the empirical literature. *Journal of Anxiety Disorders* 24(1): 1–15.

9. Ross, R.J. (2014). The changing REM sleep signature of posttraumatic stress disorder. *Sleep* 37(8): 1281–2.

10. Gieselmann, A., Ait Aoudia, M., Carr, M., Germain, A., Gorzka, R., Holzinger, B., Kleim, B., Krakow, B., Kunze, A.E., Lancee, J., et al. (2019). Aetiology and treatment of nightmare disorder: State of the art and future perspectives. *Journal of Sleep Research* 28(4): e12820.

11. Vandrey, R., Babson, K.A., Herrmann, E.S., and Bonn-Miller, M.O. (2014). Interactions between disordered sleep, post-traumatic stress disorder, and substance use disorders. *International Review of Psychiatry* 26(2): 237–47.

12. Kleim, B., Wysokowsky, J., Schmid, N., Seifritz, E., and Rasch, B. (2016). Effects of sleep after experimental trauma on intrusive emotional memories. *Sleep* 39(12): 2125–32.

19 Final words

1. Kilpatrick, D.G, Resnick, H.S., Milanak, M.E., Miller, M.W., Keyes, K.M., and Friedman, M.J. (2013). National estimates of exposure to traumatic events and PTSD prevalence using DSM-IV and DSM-5 criteria. *Journal of Traumatic Stress* 26(5): 537–47.
2. Breslau, N. The epidemiology of trauma, PTSD, and other post trauma disorders. (2009). *Trauma Violence Abuse* 10(3): 198–210.

Resources

Books

Brown, Brené, *Daring Greatly: How the Courage to be Vulnerable Transforms the*
Way We Live, Love, Parent, and Lead
Brown, Brené, *The Gifts of Imperfection*
Germer, Christopher, *The Mindful Path to Self-Compassion: Freeing Yourself from*
Destructive Thoughts and Emotions
Kabat-Zinn, Jon, *Mindfulness for Beginners*
Neff, Kristin, *Self-Compassion: The Proven Power of Being Kind to Yourself*
Smith, Spencer, and Stephen Hayes, *Get Out of Your Mind and into Your Life*
Youngson, Robin, *Time to Care: How to Love Your Patients and Your Job*

Workbooks

Evans, Wyatt R., Robyn Walser, Kent Drescher and Jacob K. Farnsworth, *Moral Injury Workbook: Acceptance and Commitment Therapy Skills for Moving beyond Shame, Anger, and Trauma to Reclaim Your Values*
Mathieu, Françoise, *Compassion Fatigue Workbook*: *Creative Tools for Transforming Compassion Fatigue and Vicarious Traumatization*, Psychosocial Stress Series 42

Places for support

Alcoholics Anonymous (UK): https://www.alcoholics-anonymous. org.uk
Alcoholics Anonymous (US): https://www.aa.org
Healthcare Workers Foundation: https://healthcareworkersfound ation. org/about-us/

Narcotics Anonymous (UK): https://ukna.org

Narcotics Anonymous (US): https://www.na.org

Second Victim: https://secondvictim.co.uk

Helplines Partnership (UK): https://helplines.org. This is a website for a directory of UK helplines.

Befrienders Worldwide: https://www.befrienders.org. This website has a tool to search by country for emotional support helplines around the world.

Helplines (UK)

Samaritans. To talk about anything that is upsetting you, you can contact Samaritans 24 hours a day, 365 days a year. You can call 116 123 (free from any phone), email jo@samaritans.org or visit some branches in person. You can also call the Samaritans Welsh Language Line on 0808 164 0123 (7pm–11pm every day).

SANEline. If you're experiencing a mental health problem or supporting someone else, you can call SANEline on 0300 304 7000 (4.30pm–10.30pm every day).

Campaign Against Living Miserably (CALM). If you identify as male, you can call the Campaign Against Living Miserably (CALM) on 0800 58 58 58 (5pm–midnight every day) or use their webchat service.

Nightline. If you're a student, you can look on the Nightline website to see if your university or college offers a night-time listening service. Nightline phone operators are all students too.

Switchboard. If you identify as gay, lesbian, bisexual or transgender, you can call Switchboard on 0300 330 0630 (10am–10pm every day), email chris@switchboard.lgbt or use their webchat service. Phone operators all identify as LGBT+.

C.A.L.L. If you live in Wales, you can call the Community Advice and Listening Line (C.A.L.L.) on 0800 132 737 (open 24/7) or you can text 'help' followed by a question to 81066.

Index